Melissa N

Color Atlas of Histopathology of the Skin

Gundula Schaumburg-Lever, M.D.

Head of the Dermatopathology Laboratory,
Department of Dermatology, Eberhard-Karls-Universität, Tübingen
Federal Republic of Germany

Walter F. Lever, M.D.

Professor Emeritus of Dermatology,
Tufts University School of Medicine
Formerly, Chairman of the Department of Dermatology,
Tufts University School of Medicine
Formerly, Lecturer on Dermatology,
Harvard Medical School,
Boston, Massachusetts

Color Atlas of Histopathology of the Skin

J. B. Lippincott Company   Philadelphia

London   Mexico City   New York   St. Louis   São Paulo   Sydney

Acquisitions Editor: Lisa A. Biello
Sponsoring Editor: Sanford J. Robinson
Manuscript Editor: Helen Ewan
Indexer: Julia Schwager
Senior Design Coordinator: Anita Curry
Designer: Paul Fry/Kate Nichols

Cover Design: Kevin M. Curry
Production Manager: Kathleen P. Dunn
Production Coordinator: George V. Gordon
Compositor: Bi-Comp, Inc.
Printer/Binder: South Sea International Press Ltd.

1   3   5   6   4   2

Library of Congress Cataloging-in-Publication Data

Schaumburg-Lever, Gundula [DATE]
    Color atlas of histopathology of the skin.

    Designed to stand alone or to be used in conjunction with: Histopathology of the skin / Walter F. Lever,
Gundula Schaumburg-Lever. 7th ed. 1988.
    Includes index.
    1. Skin—Diseases—Atlases. 2. Histology, Pathological—Atlases. I. Lever, Walter F. (Walter Fred-
erick) [DATE]   . II. Lever, Walter F. (Walter Frederick) [DATE]   Histopathology of the skin.
III. Title. [DNLM: 1. Skin Diseases—pathology—atlases. WR 17 S313c]
    RL81.S33 1988   616.5′07583   87-21431

ISBN 0-397-50832-8

Preface

This Color Atlas is conceived to stand on its own as an aid to enlarge the viewer's knowledge of dermatopathology. To derive the greatest benefit from it, it is best, however, to use it in conjunction with a textbook on dermatopathology. Naturally, we have thought foremost of our own textbook, the seventh edition of which is scheduled to appear about one year after publication of the Color Atlas. The arrangement of the photomicrographs therefore follows the chapters of our textbook.

In planning the seventh edition, it became apparent that, largely as the result of the rapid growth of immunohistochemistry, the material had grown to such an extent that it would not be possible to confine it to one volume if one wanted to include new illustrations, particularly about immunohistochemistry. Rather than having it grow into two volumes and thus making it less handy to use, we decided to add an atlas. The availability of color photography, which at one time would have made such an atlas exorbitantly expensive, was an additional incentive to work on an atlas.

In selecting the illustrations for the atlas, the two aims have been, first, choosing diagnostic microphotographs of most of the common and even less common dermatoses, provided they showed a reasonably diagnostic histologic picture; and, second, including microphotographs of immunohistochemical reactions. It should be realized that the use of monoclonal antibodies is a rapidly developing field that will greatly gain in importance for establishing diagnoses on the basis of chemical reactions rather than visual impressions, particularly in the field of tumors.

Many slides used for the photomicrographs are from our own collection, but some are from the collection of the Dermatopathology Laboratory of the Department of Dermatology at the University of Tübingen. A few have been obtained from various sources, and credit is given in such cases. The technical staff of the Dermatopathology Laboratory in Tübingen has been of great help in preparing the slides for photography. Mrs. Steitz and Mrs. Tomsky deserve special thanks.

We have also received excellent cooperation from the Medical Book Section of J. B. Lippincott Company, particularly Mr. J. Stuart Freeman, Jr.; Mr. Sanford Robinson, Developmental Editor, Medical Books; and Ms. Lisa A. Biello.

Gundula Schaumburg-Lever, M.D.
Walter F. Lever, M.D.

Abbreviations used

ABC = avidin-biotin-peroxidase complex
PAP = peroxidase-anti-peroxidase
APAAP = alkaline phosphatase anti-alkaline phosphatase

Contents

CHAPTER 3

MORPHOLOGY OF THE CELLS IN THE DERMAL INFILTRATE 15

CHAPTER 4

CONGENITAL DISEASES (GENODERMATOSES) 19

CHAPTER 5

NONINFECTIOUS VESICULAR AND BULLOUS DISEASES 25

CHAPTER 6

NONINFECTIOUS ERYTHEMATOUS, PAPULAR, AND SQUAMOUS DISEASES 37

CHAPTER 7

VASCULAR DISEASES 47

CHAPTER 8

INFLAMMATORY DISEASES OF THE EPIDERMAL APPENDAGES AND OF CARTILAGE 53

CHAPTER 9

INFLAMMATORY DISEASES DUE TO PHYSICAL AGENTS AND FOREIGN SUBSTANCES 59

CHAPTER 10

NONINFECTIOUS GRANULOMAS 65

CHAPTER 11

INFLAMMATORY DISEASES OF THE
SUBCUTANEOUS FAT 71

CHAPTER 12

ERUPTIONS DUE TO DRUGS 75

CHAPTER 13

DEGENERATIVE DISEASES 77

CHAPTER 14

BACTERIAL DISEASES 83

CHAPTER 24

METASTATIC CARCINOMA 177

CHAPTER 25

TUMORS OF FIBROUS TISSUE 185

CHAPTER 26
TUMORS OF VASCULAR TISSUE 203

CHAPTER 27
TUMORS OF FATTY, MUSCULAR, AND OSSEOUS TISSUE 219

CHAPTER 28
TUMORS OF NEURAL TISSUE 225

Color Atlas of
Histopathology
of the Skin

CHAPTER 1

Histology of the Skin

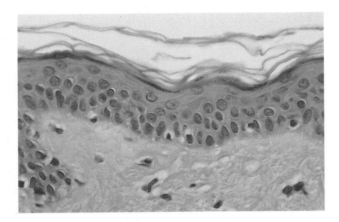

FIG. 1-1

Normal epidermis from the trunk. Four layers can be recognized: (1) basal layer, (2) squamous cell layer, (3) granular layer, (4) horny layer. The clear cells in the basal layer are melanocytes. They possess a small dark nucleus and a clear cytoplasm. (× 160)

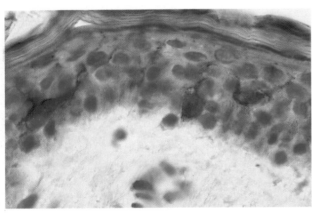

FIG. 1-2

Normal epidermis from the sole of the foot. The horny layer on the sole of the foot or the palm of the hand is considerably thicker than on any other part of the body. On the right-hand side an eccrine duct is seen to zigzag through the epidermis and the stratum corneum. (× 40)

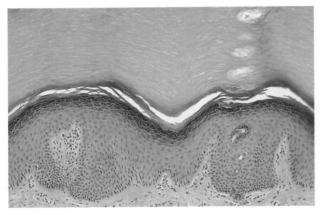

FIG. 1-3

Langerhans cells are dendritic cells in the epidermis and corium. They can be detected on frozen sections by incubating the tissue with OKT 6 or Leu 6 (this picture). The red reaction product (APAAP technique) outlines the dendritic nature of the Langerhans cells. (× 240)

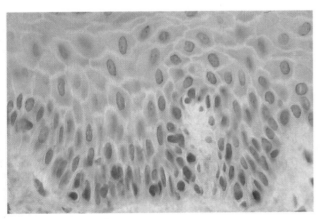

FIG. 1-4

Melanocytes can be shown by incubation with an antibody against S 100 (for further details on S 100-positive structures in the skin, refer to Figs. 2-21 through 2-24). The specific reaction product is orange (ABC technique). (× 160)

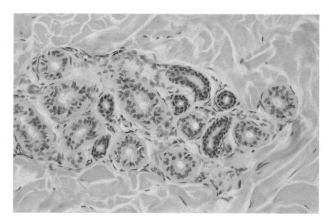

FIG. 1-5

Eccrine gland. A basal coil is shown, consisting of the secretory portion and the ductal portion of the gland. The wall of the secretory portion is composed of only one layer of secretory cells with a few myoepithelial cells wedged in at the base. The wall of the duct is composed of two layers of small, cuboidal, dark-staining cells. ($\times$ 64)

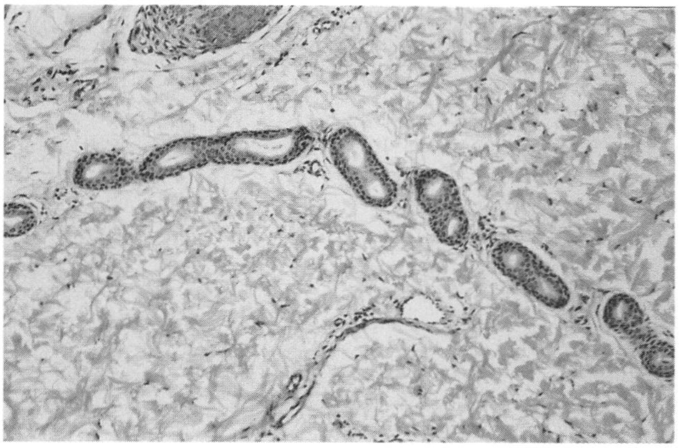

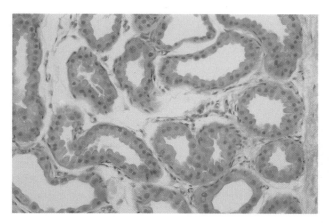

FIG. 1-6

Eccrine gland duct in the dermis. The ductal tubules are composed of two layers of small, dark-staining cells. ($\times$ 40)

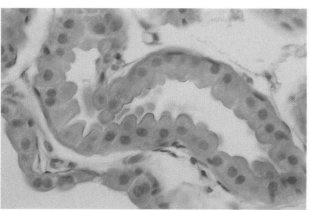

FIG. 1-7

Apocrine gland. The basal coil of the apocrine glands is located in the subcutaneous fat. The secretory portions show one layer of myoepithelial cells. Apocrine secretion can be seen on the left side of the picture. ($\times$ 64)

FIG. 1-8

Apocrine gland, higher magnification of Fig. 1.7. During apocrine secretion, the upper portions of apocrine cells are pinched off and are subsequently found in the lumen of the gland. ($\times$ 160)

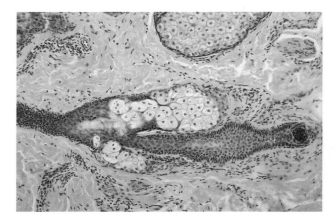

FIG. 1·9

Hair, early anagen stage. The hair is seen in its active growth stage or early anagen stage, and shows at its base a knoblike structure, the hair bulb. Attached to the hair is a sebaceous gland. (× 40)

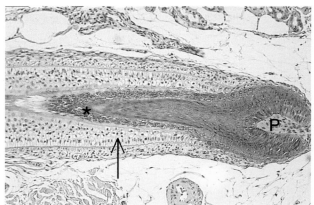

FIG. 1·10

Hair. The dermal hair papilla (P) is composed of connective tissue that protrudes into the hair bulb. The outer root sheath cells (arrow) have a clear, vacuolated cytoplasm owing to the presence of glycogen. The inner root sheath (asterisk) keratinizes by means of trichohyalin granules, which stain eosinophilic. (× 40)

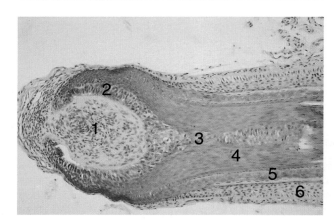

FIG. 1·11

Hair. Lower portion of an anagen hair follicle consisting of the following parts: (1) papilla, (2) matrix, (3) medulla, (4) cortex, (5) inner root sheath, (6) outer root sheath. (× 64)

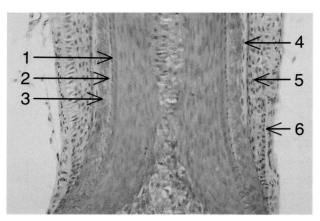

FIG. 1·12

Hair. The various linings of the hair can be recognized: (1) hair cuticle, (2) inner root sheath cuticle, (3) multiple Huxley layers, (4) a single Henle's layer, (5) outer root sheath, (6) glassy or vitreous layer. (× 160)

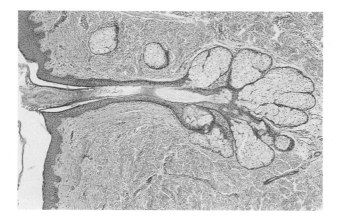

FIG. 1-13

The **sebaceous gland** consists of several lobules leading into a common excretory duct composed of stratified squamous epithelium. Each sebaceous lobule possesses a peripheral layer of cuboidal, deeply basophilic cells that contain no lipid droplets. ($\times$ 13)

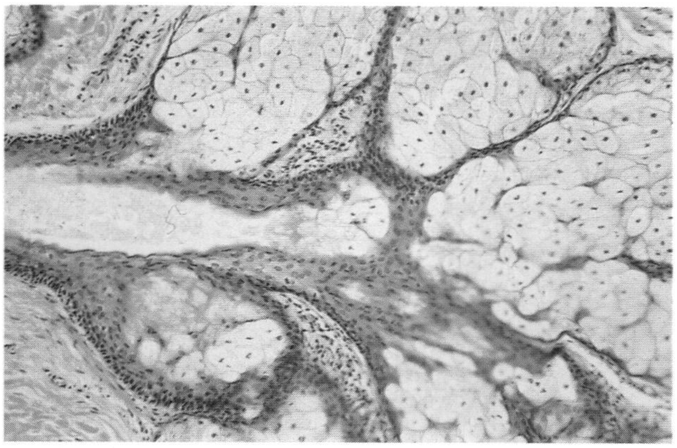

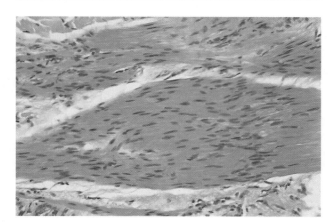

FIG. 1-14

Sebaceous gland. The nucleus of a sebaceous gland cell is centrally located. In the portion of the lobule located closest to the duct, the cells disintegrate. Amorphous material is seen in the duct. ($\times$ 40)

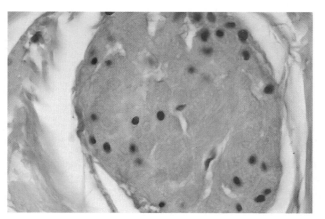

FIG. 1-15

A **smooth muscle,** *i.e.,* arrector pilorum, is characterized by the lack of striation and by elongated nuclei located in the center of the cell. ($\times$ 64)

FIG. 1-16

Smooth muscle. On cross section, the central location of the nucleus can be seen. ($\times$ 240)

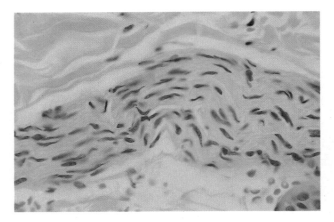

FIG. 1-17

Unmyelinated (autonomic) nerve. Nerves are composed of neuraxons and Schwann cells (sheath cells or neurilemmal cells). The Schwann cells consist of elongated nuclei and long, wavy processes. (× 160)

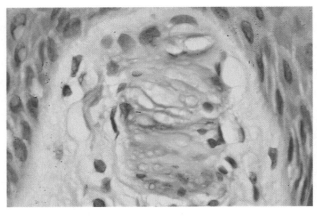

FIG. 1-18

A **Meissner corpuscle** is located in the papilla of the fingertip. A Meissner corpuscle possesses a capsule composed of several layers of flattened Schwann cells. Inside the corpuscle they are arranged transverse to the long axis of the corpuscle. The section has been incubated with a monoclonal antibody against neurofilaments (APAAP technique). Neurofilaments are part of the cytoskeleton of a neuron. (× 240)

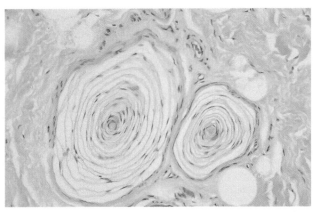

FIG. 1-19

Vater-Pacini corpuscles are nerve end-organs located in the subcutis. They consist of a stalk with a single thick nerve that is surrounded by a thick capsule. The capsule consists of concentric, loosely arranged lamellae. (× 64)

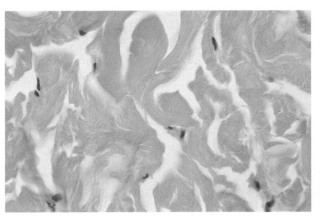

FIG. 1-20

Collagen fibers are arranged in bundles that extend in various directions. A small number of fibroblasts are interspersed between the collagen bundles. Collagen is eosinophilic. (× 160)

CHAPTER 2

Laboratory
Methods

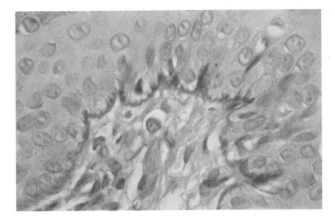

FIG. 2-1

The **periodic acid-Schiff (PAS)** stain demonstrates the presence of certain polysaccharides, particularly glycogen and mucoprotein containing neutral mucopolysaccharides, by staining them red. The PAS outlines the subepidermal basement membrane zone as a homogenous band. (× 240)

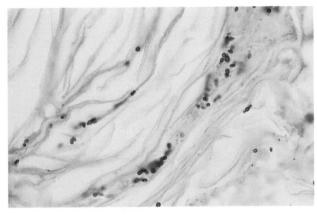

FIG. 2-2

The **PAS stain** is also used to demonstrate the presence of fungi in tissue. Since the cell walls of fungi are composed of a mixture of cellulose and chitin, and thus contain polysaccharides, all fungi stain red. (× 240)

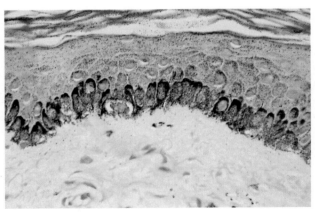

FIG. 2-3

The **Fontana-Masson** (ammoniated silver nitrate) stain demonstrates the presence of melanin by staining it black. (× 160)

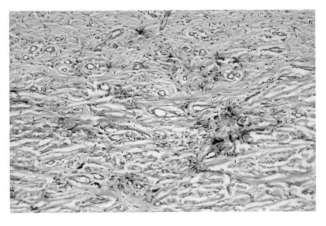

FIG. 2-4

Perls' potassium ferrocyanide stain demonstrates the presence of hemosiderin by staining it blue. (× 40)

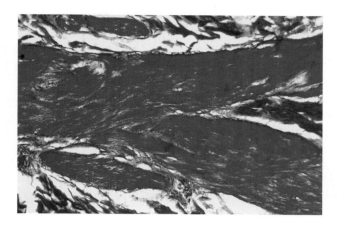

FIG. 2-5

Masson's trichrome stain stains muscles (this picture), nuclei, and nerves dark red. (× 40)

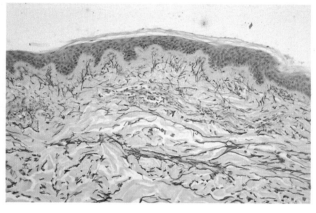

FIG. 2-6

Pinkus' acid orcein stains elastic fibers dark brown, as shown on this micrograph. The section has been counterstained with methylene green. (× 40)

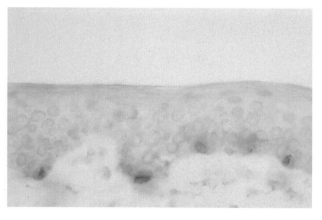

FIG. 2-7

The **dopa reaction** requires fresh, unfixed tissue. Frozen sections are incubated with 3,4-dihydroxyphenylalanine (called dopa). Tyrosinase, present in melanocytes, changes the colorless dopa of the staining solution through oxidation into dopa-melanin, which is black (this picture). (× 160)

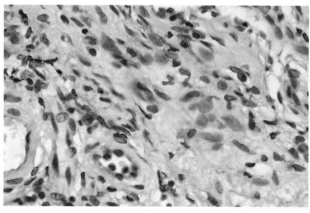

FIG. 2-8

Naphthol AS-D chloracetate esterase is used to outline mast cells (this picture) or granulocytic myelocytes. It can be used on paraffin sections. (× 160)

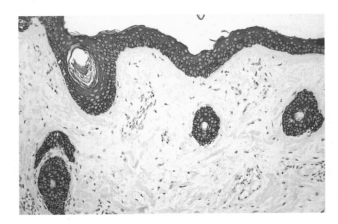

FIG. 2-9

Keratin, one of the cytoskeletal filaments. The section has been incubated with a monoclonal antibody against keratin. Keratin is present in the epidermis and the epidermal appendages. Incubation with anti-keratin is useful for the detection of carcinomas. APAAP technique. (× 40)

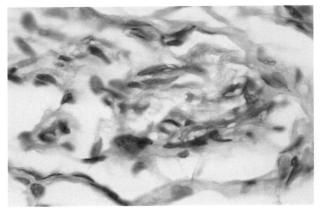

FIG. 2-10

Neurofilaments, one of the cytoskeletal filaments. The section has been incubated with a monoclonal antibody against neurofilaments, which have been found in neurons only. This antibody is helpful in identifying undifferentiated tumors of neuronal origin. APAAP technique. (× 240)

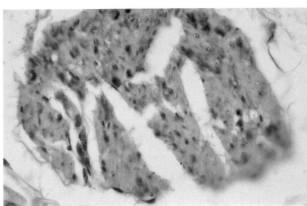

FIG. 2-11

Desmin, one of the cytoskeletal filaments. The monoclonal antibody against desmin reacts with both smooth and striated muscle and helps to identify tumors of muscular origin. ABC technique. (× 160)

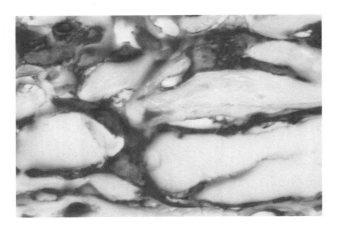

FIG. 2-12

Vimentin, one of the cytoskeletal filaments. The monoclonal antibody against vimentin identifies cells of mesenchymal origin, *i.e.,* fibroblasts (this picture). Melanocytes also contain vimentin. APAAP technique. (× 400)

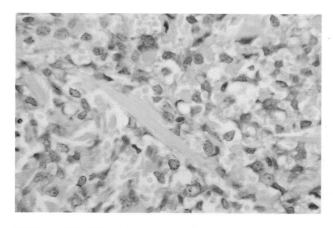

FIG. 2-13

Lysozyme staining of macrophages. Incubation with a polyclonal antibody against lysozyme. Lysozyme is predominantly found in macrophages with active phagocytosis. ABC technique. (× 160)

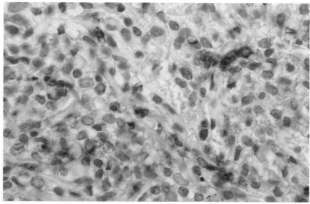

FIG. 2-14

Chymotrypsin staining of macrophages. Incubation with a polyclonal antibody against alpha$_1$-antichymotrypsin, another marker for macrophages. ABC technique. (× 160)

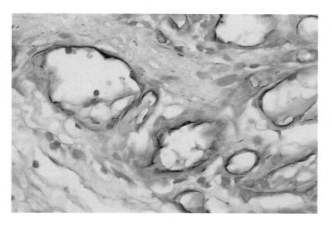

FIG. 2-15

Ulex europaeus I staining of endothelial cells. Incubation with the lectin Ulex europaeus agglutinin I, which reacts specifically with α-L-fucose. Fucose is present in endothelial cells, and therefore Ulex europaeus I can be used as an endothelial marker (see Figs. 26-2, 26-31, 26-32, 26-39, and 26-40). Ulex works well on paraffin sections. PAP technique. (× 160)

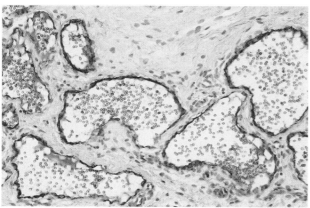

FIG. 2-16

Factor VIII-related antigen staining of endothelial cells. Incubation with a monoclonal antibody against factor VIII-related antigen, another marker for endothelial cells. This antibody is not as reliable in paraffin sections as Ulex europaeus, but works well on frozen sections. APAAP technique. (× 64)

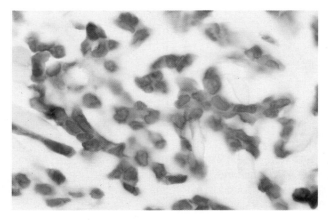

FIG. 2-17

Lambda chains staining of plasma cells. Incubation with a monoclonal antibody against lambda chains that are present in plasma cells. After preincubation with pronase, lambda chains can be revealed. ABC technique. (× 240)

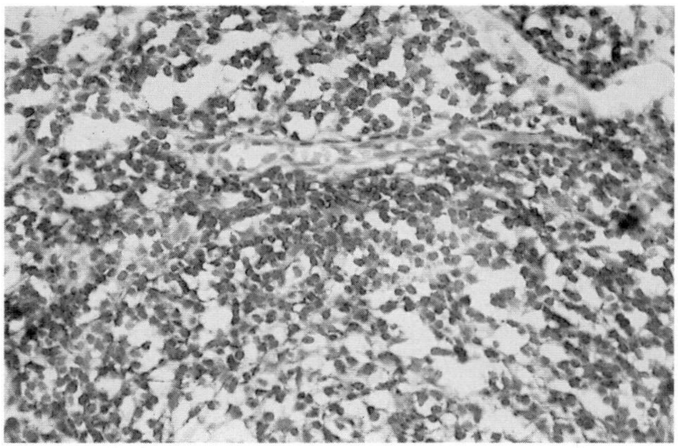

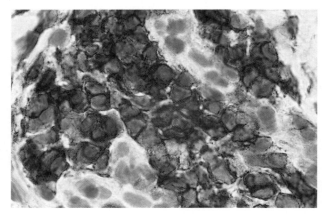

FIG. 2-18

Leukocyte common antigen staining of lymphocytes. Incubation with a monoclonal antibody against leukocyte common antigen. This antibody works on paraffin sections and is useful for the differential diagnosis between an anaplastic lymphoma and an anaplastic carcinoma. PAP technique. (× 64)

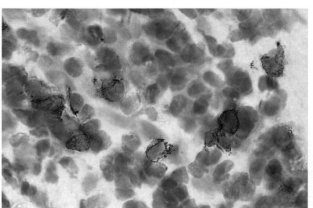

FIG. 2-19

Leu 3a staining of T helper cells. Incubation with the monoclonal antibody Leu 3a identifies T helper cells in frozen sections. APAAP technique. (× 240)

FIG. 2-20

Leu 2a staining of T suppressor cells. Incubation with the monoclonal antibody Leu 2a identifies T suppressor cells in frozen sections. APAAP technique. (× 240)

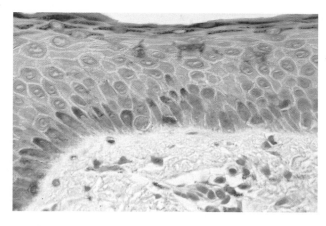

FIG. 2-21

S 100 protein staining of melanocytes and Langerhans cells. Polyclonal antibody against S 100 protein identifies melanocytes and Langerhans cells in the epidermis. The antibody can be used on paraffin sections. ABC technique. (× 160)

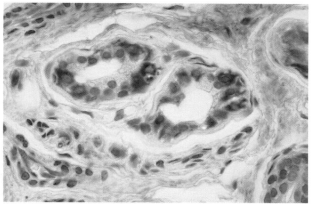

FIG. 2-22

S 100 protein staining of eccrine gland cells. Antibody against S 100 protein reacts with eccrine gland cells, but not with eccrine ducts. ABC technique. (× 160)

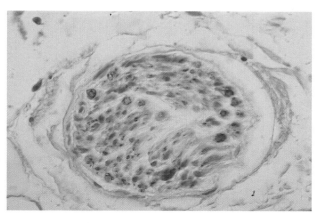

FIG. 2-23

S 100 protein staining of Schwann cells. S 100 protein is also present in Schwann cells of nerves. ABC technique. (× 160)

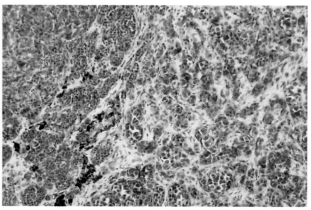

FIG. 2-24

S 100 protein staining of melanoma cells. Antibody against S 100 protein is often used to identify melanoma cells (this picture). ABC technique. (× 40)

CHAPTER 3

Morphology
of the Cells
in the Dermal
Infiltrate

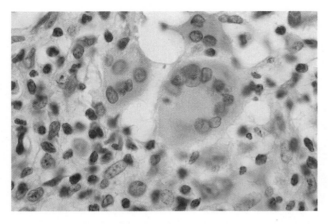

FIG. 3-1

Two **foreign body giant cells** can be seen. In the cell on the right side, the nuclei are arranged along the periphery in a semicircular fashion (Langhans type of a giant cell), whereas in the giant cell on the left side, the nuclei are distributed in clusters. (× 240)

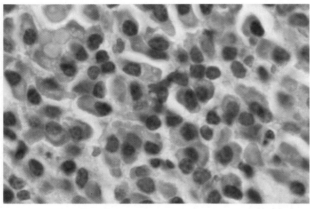

FIG. 3-2

Plasma cells have abundant cytoplasm and an eccentrically placed round nucleus. The nuclei show regularly distributed chromatin particles along their membrane, which give the nuclei a cartwheel appearance. (× 240)

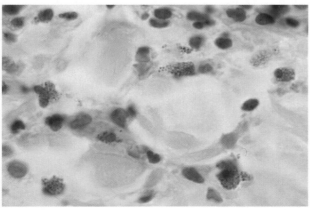

FIG. 3-3

Melanophages are macrophages that have phagocytized melanin. (× 240)

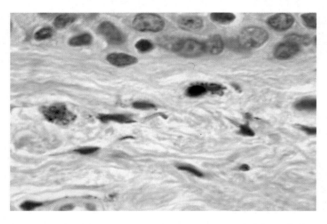

FIG. 3-4

Eosinophilic granulocytes are characterized by the presence of eosinophilic granules in the cytoplasm. (× 240)

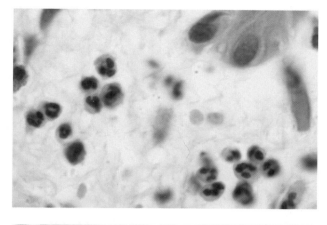

FIG. 3-5

Neutrophilic granulocytes have a lobulated nucleus consisting of several segments that are connected by narrow bridges of nucleoplasm. (× 240)

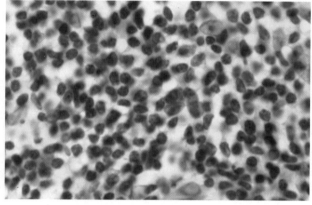

FIG. 3-6

Lymphocytes possess a relatively small, round nucleus that appears deeply basophilic because of the presence of numerous chromatin particles. They have only a narrow rim of cytoplasm, which is hardly visible. (× 160)

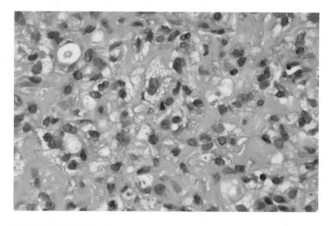

FIG. 3-7

Foam cells are macrophages that have accumulated lipids in their cytoplasm. (× 160)

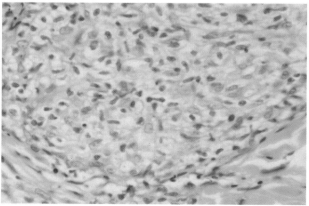

FIG. 3-8

Epithelioid cells arise from macrophages. They possess a large, oval, pale, vesicular nucleus and abundant, ill-defined, slightly eosinophilic cytoplasm. This picture shows an epithelioid tubercle with only a few lymphocytes at the periphery, as seen, for example, in sarcoidosis. (× 160)

CHAPTER 4

Congenital Diseases (Genodermatoses)

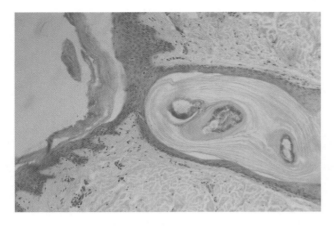

FIG. 4-1

Ichthyosis vulgaris. The epidermis shows a moderate degree of hyperkeratosis with a thin or absent granular layer. The hyperkeratosis extends into the hair follicles, resulting in a large keratotic plug. (× 16)

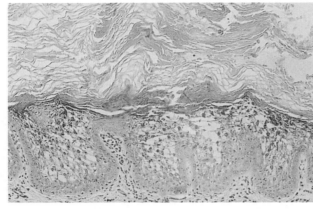

FIG. 4-2

Epidermolytic hyperkeratosis is seen in bullous congenital ichthyosiform erythroderma. Evident are (1) clear spaces around the nuclei in the upper stratum spinosum and in the stratum granulosum, (2) indistinct cellular boundaries, (3) a thickened granular layer containing an increased number of keratohyaline granules, (4) hyperkeratosis. (× 40)

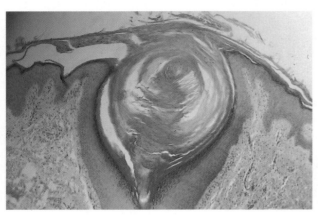

FIG. 4-3

Keratosis pilaris. A dilated infundibulum of a hair follicle is seen that is filled with a keratotic plug. (× 40)

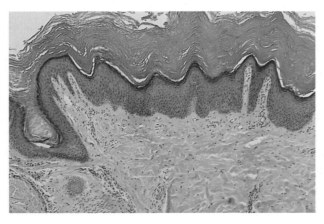

FIG. 4-4

Erythrokeratodermia variabilis. The histologic changes are nonspecific. They consist of hyperkeratosis with moderate papillomatosis and acanthosis. The granular layer appears normal. (× 10)

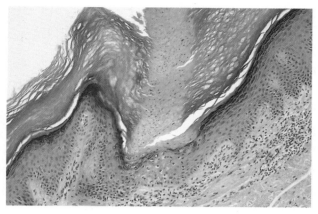

FIG. 4-5

Porokeratosis Mibelli. The epidermis shows a keratin-filled invagination, which extends deeply downward at an angle. In the center of this invagination a parakeratotic column rises, the so-called cornoid lamella. (× 40)

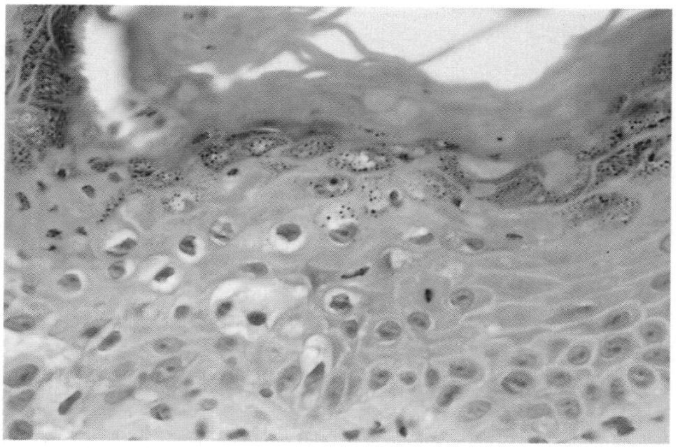

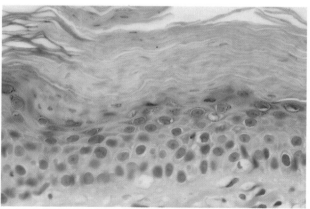

FIG. 4-6

Porokeratosis Mibelli. The parakeratotic column shows at the base epidermal cells that have pyknotic nuclei with perinuclear edema. (× 160)

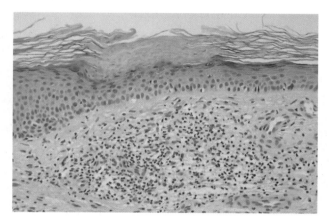

FIG. 4-7

Disseminated superficial actinic porokeratosis. The central invagination is shallow. The parakeratotic column consists of homogeneous cells rather than the basketweave pattern seen in the surrounding orthokeratotic stratum corneum. (× 64)

FIG. 4-8

Disseminated superficial actinic porokeratosis. The central furrow is shallow. The perinuclear vacuolization is less pronounced than in porokeratosis of Mibelli. (× 160)

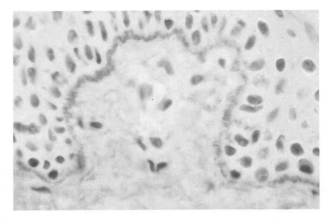

FIG. 4-9

Epidermolysis bullosa acquisita. The section has been incubated with protein A, which binds specifically with the Fc fragment of IgG. In this disease, an autoimmune disorder, a linear band of IgG is seen beneath the electron microscopic basal lamina. ABC technique. ($\times$ 240)

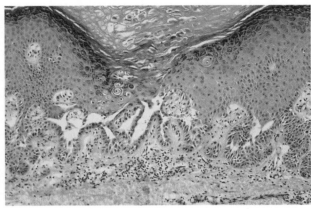

FIG. 4-10

Keratosis follicularis (Darier's disease). The characteristic changes are (1) a peculiar form of dyskeratosis, resulting in corps ronds and grains; (2) suprabasal acantholysis, leading to the formation of suprabasal clefts; (3) irregular upward proliferation into the lacunae of papillae lined with a single layer of basal cells. ($\times$ 40)

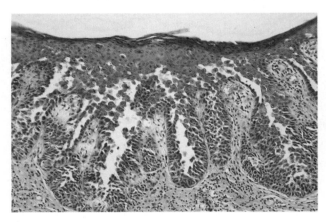

FIG. 4-11

Familial benign pemphigus (Hailey-Hailey disease). Acantholysis has affected large portions of the epidermis. The cells of the detached epidermis show only slight separation from one another because a few intact intercellular bridges still hold them loosely together. This quite typical feature gives the detached epidermis the appearance of a dilapidated brick wall. ($\times$ 40)

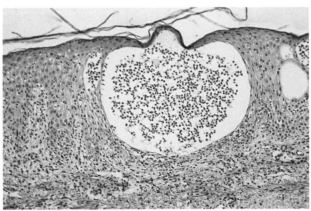

FIG. 4-12

Incontinentia pigmenti, vesicular stage. The vesicles arise in the epidermis and are associated with spongiosis. Numerous eosinophils and mononuclear cells are present in the vesicles as well as in the epidermis and dermis. ($\times$ 40)

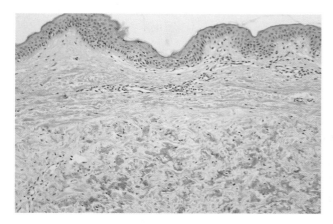

FIG. 4-13

Pseudoxanthoma elasticum, H&E stain. In the middle and lower dermis the elastic fibers appear swollen and irregularly clumped. They stain faintly basophilic because of their calcium content. (× 40)

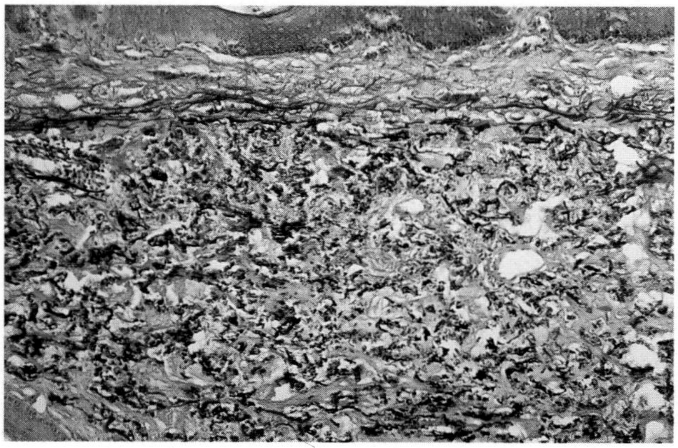

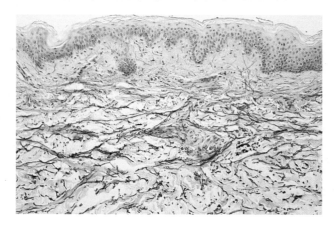

FIG. 4-14

Pseudoxanthoma elasticum, elastic tissue stain. The elastic fibers in the upper portion of the dermis have a normal appearance. In the lower portion they show degeneration. Verhoeff stain stains elastic fibers black. (× 40)

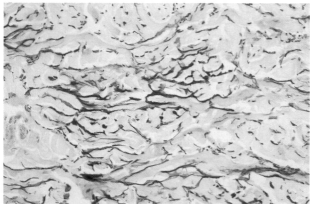

FIG. 4-15

Nevus elasticus, elastic tissue stain. The elastic fibers are increased in number and size without showing signs of degeneration. Resorcin-fuchsin stain stains elastic fibers dark red. (× 40)

FIG. 4-16

Nevus elasticus, elastic tissue stain, higher magnification. The elastic fibers are increased in number, but otherwise, they appear normal. (× 64)

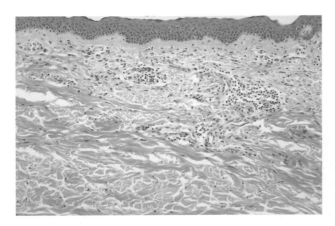

FIG. 4-17

Urticaria pigmentosa, maculopapular type, H&E stain. The upper dermis shows a perivascular infiltrate of mononuclear cells, some of which are mast cells. (× 40)

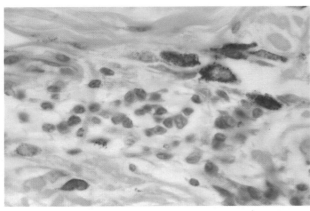

FIG. 4-18

Urticaria pigmentosa, maculopapular type, Giemsa stain. The mast cells are spindle shaped. The mast cell granules stain metachromatically with Giemsa. (× 240)

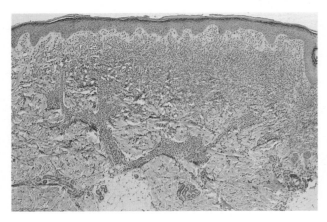

FIG. 4-19

Urticaria pigmentosa, plaque type, H&E stain. The mast cells lie closely packed in the upper dermis. (× 10)

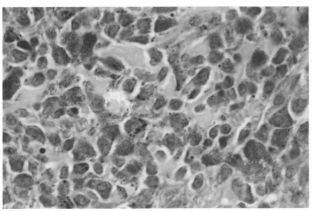

FIG. 4-20

Urticaria pigmentosa, plaque type, Giemsa stain. The mast cells appear as cuboidal cells. (× 240)

C H A P T E R 5

Noninfectious Vesicular and Bullous Diseases

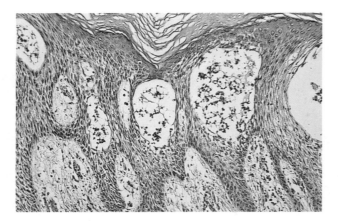

FIG. 5-1

Acute dermatitis. Numerous intraepidermal vesicles can be seen, and there is pronounced intraepidermal edema (spongiosis). The vesicles contain mononuclear cells. (× 40)

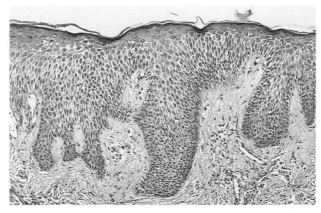

FIG. 5-2

Subacute dermatitis. There is moderate acanthosis and pronounced spongiosis. Intraepidermal vesicles may or may not be present. (× 40)

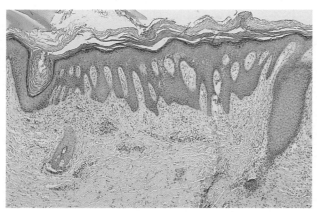

FIG. 5-3

Chronic dermatitis. There is moderate to marked acanthosis with elongation of the rete ridges. The stratum corneum is hyperkeratotic. In the upper dermis a perivascular infiltrate of mononuclear cells can be seen. (× 13)

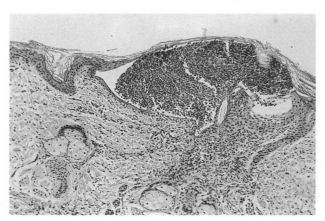

FIG. 5-4

Erythema toxicum neonatorum. A pustule filled with eosinophils can be seen in a follicular location. The outer root sheath beneath the pustule is filled with eosinophils. (× 10)

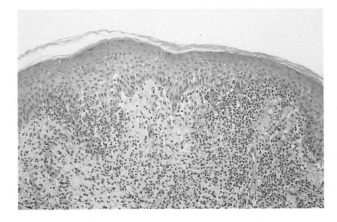

FIG. 5-5

Pemphigus vulgaris. In rare instances eosinophils invade the epidermis before acantholysis has become evident. This has been referred to as eosinophilic spongiosis. (× 40)

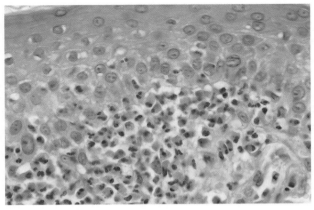

FIG. 5-6

Pemphigus vulgaris. Higher magnification of eosinophilic spongiosis. Eosinophils have accumulated beneath the epidermis and have started to invade the epidermis. Acantholysis is not yet evident. (× 160)

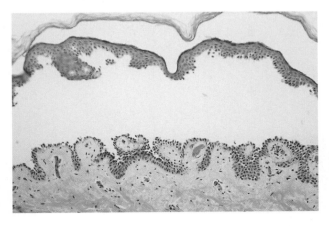

FIG. 5-7

Pemphigus vulgaris. A suprabasal blister has formed. A few acantholytic cells can be seen in the blister cavity. Because of regeneration, the base of the blister consists of more than one layer in several areas. (× 40)

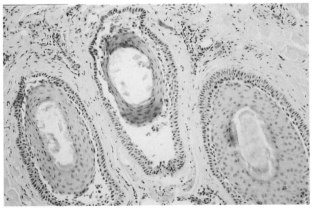

FIG. 5-8

Pemphigus vulgaris. Acantholysis is not limited to the epidermis, but also occurs in the outer root sheath of hair follicles. (× 40)

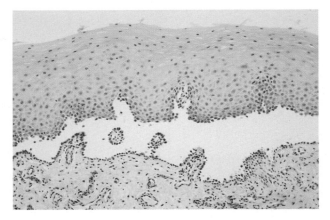

FIG. 5-9

Pemphigus vulgaris, oral mucosa. The blister is located in a suprabasal location. There is only slight inflammation beneath the bulla. (× 40)

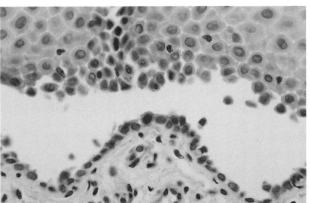

FIG. 5-10

Pemphigus vulgaris, oral mucosa. The base of the blister is formed by the basal cells, which remain attached to the dermis like a row of tombstones. A few single acantholytic cells can be seen in the blister cavity. (× 240)

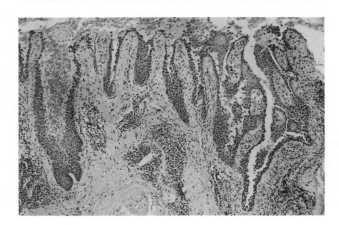

FIG. 5-11

Pemphigus vegetans, early lesion. The epidermis shows marked downward proliferation of epithelial strands and formation of villi. Within the intraepidermal clefts, acantholytic cells can be seen. (× 16)

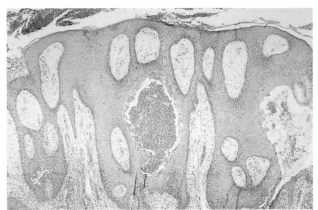

FIG. 5-12

Pemphigus vegetans, late lesion. The section was obtained from a verrucous lesion and shows considerable acanthosis and formation of intraepidermal abscesses consisting of eosinophils. (× 16)

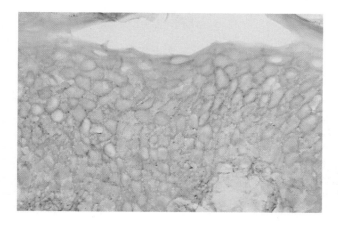

FIG. 5·13

Pemphigus vulgaris, direct immunoperoxidase method. The section was incubated with protein A, which binds specifically with the Fc portion of IgG. *In vivo* bound IgG is found in the intercellular space. The specific reaction product is brown. ABC technique. (× 160)

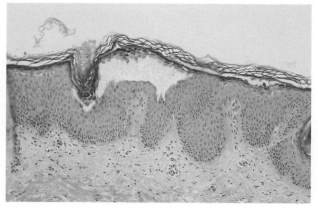

FIG. 5·14

Pemphigus foliaceus. Acantholysis occurs in the granular layer or just beneath it, leading to the formation of a cleft in a superficial location. (× 40)

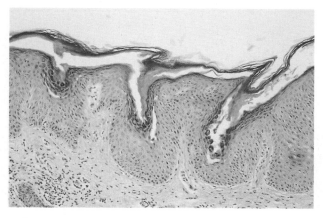

FIG. 5·15

Pemphigus foliaceus, very early lesion. Three small clefts have formed beneath the granular layer. The acantholytic granular cells appear shrunken and hyperchromatic. (× 40)

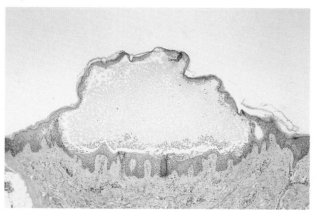

FIG. 5·16

Pemphigus foliaceus. A blister has formed in the upper epidermis. (× 64)

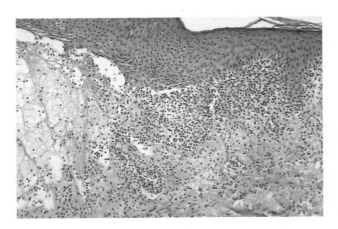

FIG. 5-17

Bullous pemphigoid, inflamed lesion. A bulla on the left side has arisen by detachment of the epidermis from the dermis. The epidermis at the roof of the blister appears intact. The blister contains strands of fibrin and eosinophils. Adjacent to the blister, accumulations of eosinophils can be seen in the papillae. ($\times$ 40)

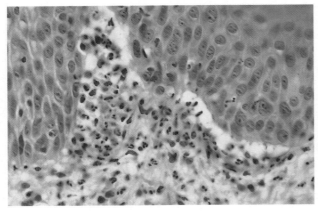

FIG. 5-18

Bullous pemphigoid, inflamed lesion. An intrapapillary abscess predominantly consisting of eosinophils, but also containing some neutrophils, can be seen. On the right side a small cleft has formed between the epidermis and the dermis. ($\times$ 160)

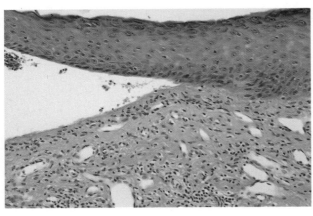

FIG. 5-19

Bullous pemphigoid, edge of a bulla, noninflamed lesion. The blister does not contain any fibrin or eosinophils. The dermis contains a diffuse infiltration of mononuclear cells. ($\times$ 64)

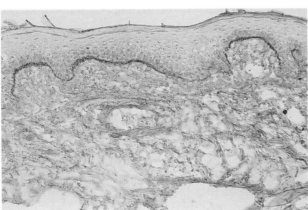

FIG. 5-20

Bullous pemphigoid, direct immunoperoxidase method. The section has been incubated with anti-IgG. A linear band of IgG (brown reaction product) can be seen at the dermal-epidermal junction. ABC technique. ($\times$ 30)

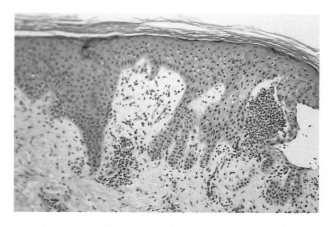

FIG. 5-21

Dermatitis herpetiformis. The biopsy is taken from the edge of a blister. Next to the edge of the blister a papillary microabscess consisting of neutrophils can be seen. (× 40)

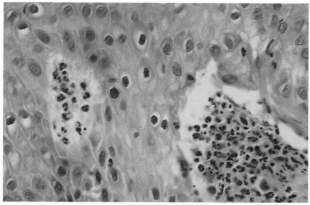

FIG. 5-22

Dermatitis herpetiformis, higher magnification. The microabscess predominantly consists of neutrophils. (× 160)

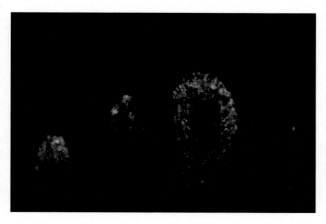

FIG. 5-23

Dermatitis herpetiformis, direct immunofluorescence. Granular deposits of IgA are seen at the tips of the papillae. (Courtesy by K. Sönnichsen, M.D.) (× 40)

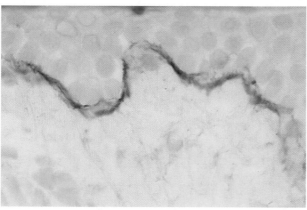

FIG. 5-24

Linear IgA dermatosis. A linear band of IgA deposits can be seen at the dermal-epidermal junction. The IgA deposits in this case were found directly beneath the basal lamina when immunoelectron microscopy was performed. ABC technique. (× 240)

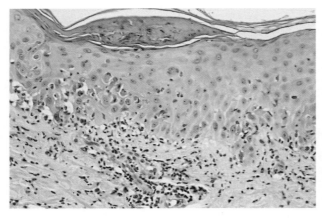

FIG. 5-25

Erythema multiforme, mixed dermal-epidermal type. A mononuclear infiltrate is present along the dermal-epidermal border. The basal cells on the left side show hydropic degeneration. The epidermis contains numerous scattered individually necrotic keratinocytes showing a strongly eosinophilic cytoplasm. ($\times$ 40)

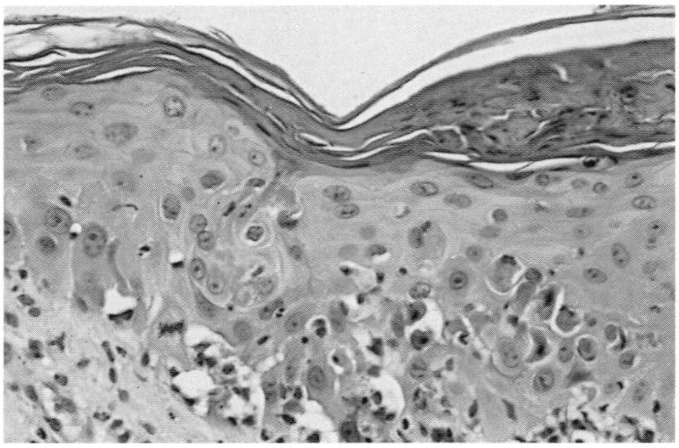

FIG. 5-26

Erythema multiforme, mixed dermal-epidermal type, higher magnification. The basal cells show hydropic degeneration. Within the epidermis numerous scattered individually necrotic keratinocytes can be seen. They stain strongly eosinophilic and have either pyknotic nuclei or no nuclei. ($\times$ 64)

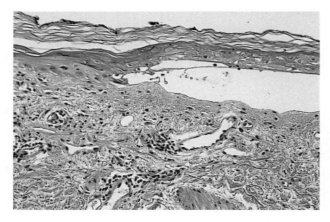

FIG. 5-27

Erythema multiforme, epidermal type. On the right-hand side the epidermis is necrotic. This can be seen in toxic epidermal necrolysis. The dermal changes consist only of a mild mononuclear infiltrate around the superficial blood vessels. ($\times$ 40)

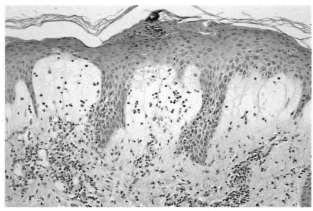

FIG. 5-28

Erythema multiforme, dermal type. The upper dermis shows marked edema, resulting in subepidermal blisters. A fairly pronounced perivascular infiltrate consisting of mononuclear cells is present in the dermis. ($\times$ 40)

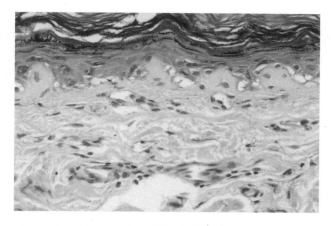

FIG. 5-29

Graft-versus-host disease, acute phase. The basal cells show pronounced hydropic degeneration. (× 64)

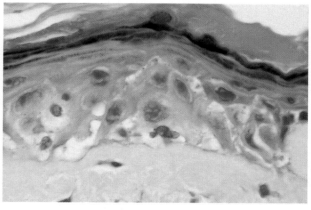

FIG. 5-30

Graft-versus-host disease, higher magnification of Fig. 5-29. The basal cells show pronounced hydropic degeneration, and there is some spongiosis in the epidermis. (× 240)

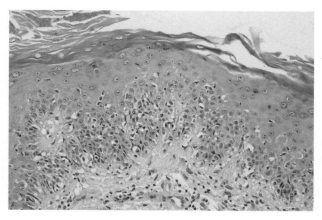

FIG. 5-31

Graft-versus-host disease, acute phase. In addition to hydropic degeneration of the basal cells and some spongiosis, dyskeratosis of epidermal cells can be seen. (× 64)

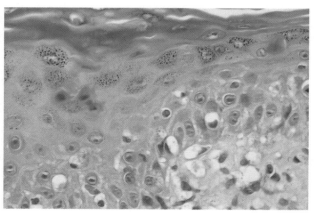

FIG. 5-32

Graft-versus-host-disease, acute phase. Within the epidermis, groups of dyskeratotic keratinocytes can be seen. There is some spongiosis and hydropic degeneration of the basal cells. (× 240)

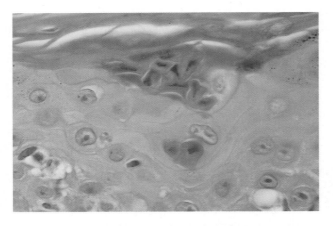

FIG. 5-33

Graft-versus-host disease, acute phase. Groups of dyskeratotic keratinocytes can be seen. (× 240)

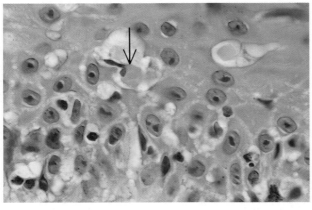

FIG. 5-34

Graft-versus-host disease, acute phase. A necrotic keratinocyte is seen in association with a satellite lymphocyte (arrow). This association is referred to as satellite cell necrosis. (× 240)

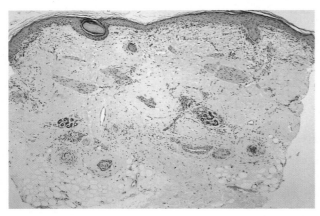

FIG. 5-35

Graft-versus-host disease, chronic phase. At low magnification, sclerosis can be seen, resembling scleroderma. The dermis shows thickened and hyalinized collagen extending into the subcutaneous fat. The eccrine glands are surrounded by thickened collagen rather than by fat cells. (× 16)

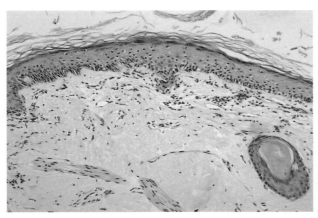

FIG. 5-36

Graft-versus-host disease, chronic phase, higher magnification of Fig. 5-35. The biopsy was taken from the scalp. The hair follicles, except for one, have been replaced by sclerotic collagen. (× 40)

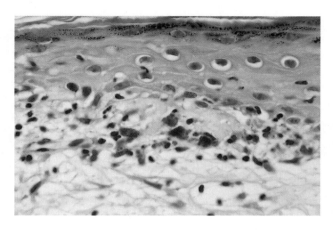

FIG. 5-37

Graft-versus-host disease, chronic phase, higher magnification of Fig. 5-35. A necrotic keratinocyte is seen in association with a satellite lymphocyte. There is cell necrosis in the basal layer and pigmentary incontinence in the upper dermis. (× 160)

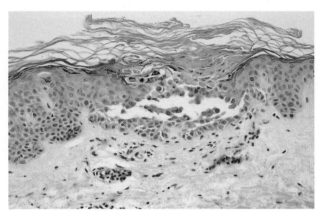

FIG. 5-38

Graft-versus-host disease, chronic phase, higher magnification of Fig. 5-35. The eccrine glands are surrounded by collagen instead of by fat cells. (× 160)

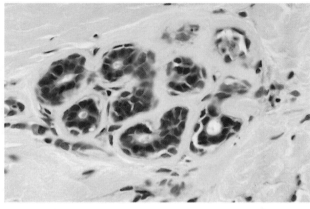

FIG. 5-39

Transient acantholytic disease. Within the epidermis, localized acantholysis can be seen. The pattern resembles keratosis follicularis (Darier's disease) with "grains" in the granular layer. (× 64)

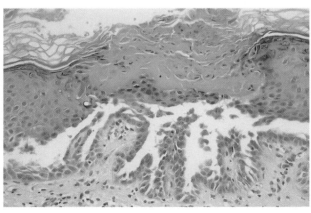

FIG. 5-40

Transient acantholytic disease. The suprabasal acantholysis resembles pemphigus vulgaris. Within the blister cavity, groups of acantholytic cells can be seen. (× 64)

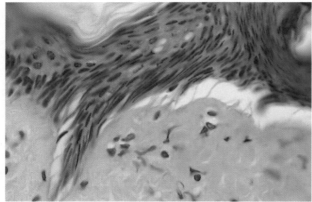

FIG. 5-41

Artifact caused by electrodesiccation. A subepidermal cleft has formed. The nuclei and the cytoplasmic processes of the keratinocytes of the lower half of the epidermis have been stretched in the same direction and resemble goat whiskers. (× 160)

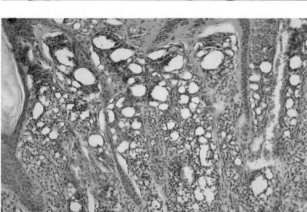

FIG. 5-42

Artifact due to freezing of the tissue during transport. The tissue resembles Swiss cheese, owing to freezing artifact. This can be avoided by diluting formaldehyde with 50% ethanol instead of distilled water during the cold season. (× 40)

CHAPTER 6

Noninfectious Erythematous, Papular, and Squamous Diseases

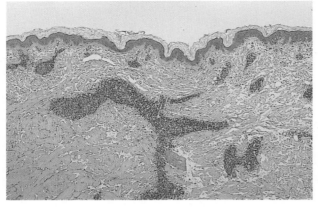

FIG. 6-1

Erythema annulare centrifugum. A cellular infiltrate in a fairly sharply demarcated perivascular coat sleeve-like arrangement is present in the middle and lower dermis. (× 13)

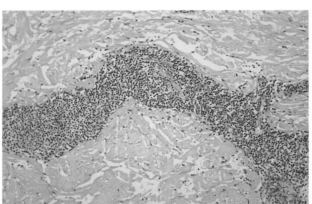

FIG. 6-2

Erythema annulare centrifugum, higher magnification. A thick perivascular sleeve of mononuclear cells, largely lymphocytes, is seen. (× 40)

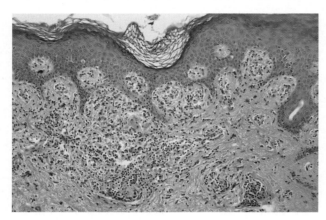

FIG. 6-3

Erythema dyschromicum perstans. The basal cell layer of the epidermis has disappeared. The upper dermis shows a moderate infiltrate of lymphocytes, macrophages, and melanophages. (× 40)

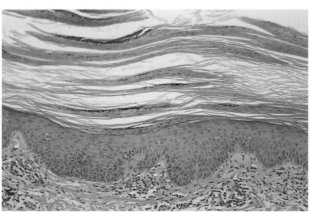

FIG. 6-4

Psoriasis, early lesion. The stratum corneum shows scattered parakeratotic mounds within an otherwise orthokeratotic stratum corneum. Some of the parakeratotic mounds show degenerated neutrophils in their summit. (× 40)

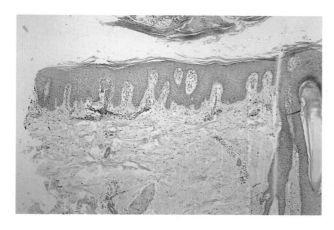

FIG. 6-5

Psoriasis. The rete ridges show regular elongation, with thickening in the lower portions. The papillae are elongated. (× 16)

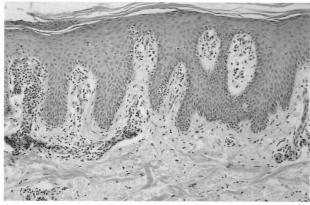

FIG. 6-6

Psoriasis, higher magnification of Fig. 6-4. The epidermis shows acanthosis. The rete ridges are elongated and thickened. The dermal papillae are elongated and edematous. (× 40)

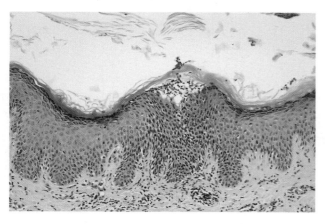

FIG. 6-7

Psoriasis. In the uppermost portion of the spinous layer a minute spongiform pustule of Kogoj can be seen. A spongiform pustule consists of an accumulation of neutrophils intermingled with keratinocytes. This spongiform pustule is highly diagnostic for psoriasis. (× 40)

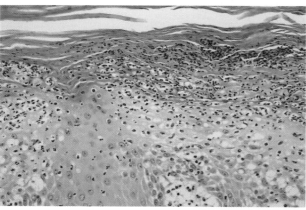

FIG. 6-8

Psoriasis, pustular. Another spongiform pustule consisting of keratinocytes intermingled with neutrophils. Aggregates of neutrophils are seen within interstices of a spongelike network formed by degenerated and thinned epidermal cells. (× 64)

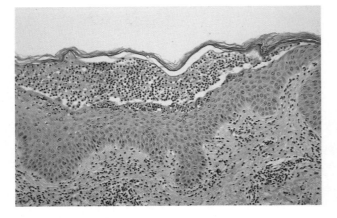

FIG. 6-9

Psoriasis, pustular. Within the stratum corneum a Munro abscess can be seen. It consists of accumulations of pyknotic nuclei of neutrophils that have migrated there from capillaries in the papillae through the suprapapillary epidermis. (× 40)

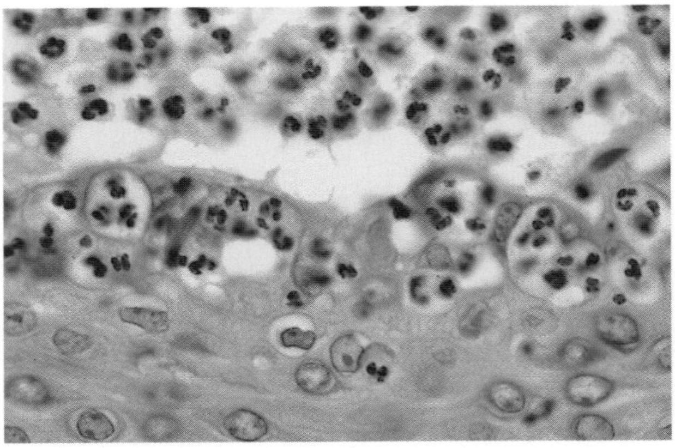

FIG. 6-10

Psoriasis, pustular, higher magnification of Fig. 6-9. Under the Munro abscess, neutrophils are seen within the interstices of a spongelike network formed by degenerated and thinned epidermal cells. (× 240)

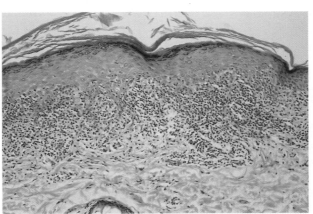

FIG. 6-11

Psoriasis. Incubation with Ulex europaeus agglutinin I, an endothelial marker, shows that in psoriasis, all capillaries are elongated, widened, and tortuous. PAP technique. (× 30)

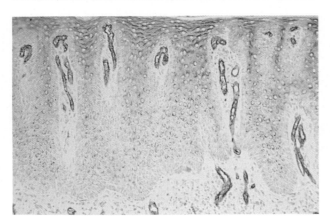

FIG. 6-12

Lichen planus, early lesion. There are hyperkeratosis, focal hypergranulosis, and acanthosis. The basal layer has been invaded by the bandlike inflammatory infiltrate and appears "wiped out." (× 40)

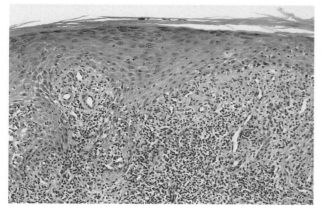

FIG. 6-13

Lichen planus. The stratum granulosum shows irregular thickening. On the left side the rete ridges show irregular elongation, and they are pointed at the lower end, giving them a sawtooth appearance. (× 40)

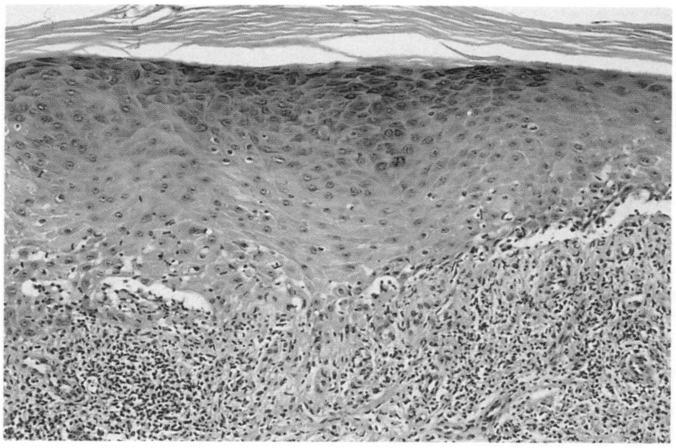

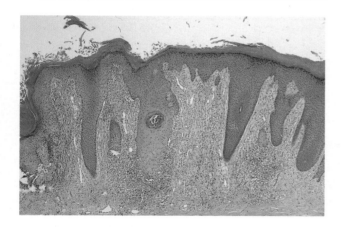

FIG. 6-14

Lichen planus. The stratum granulosum is irregularly thickened. Small areas of separation are seen between the epidermis and the dermis, and these are referred to as Max Joseph spaces. The separation is the result of damage of the basal cells. (× 40)

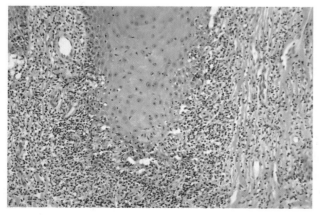

FIG. 6-15

Lichen planus, hypertrophic form. The lesion shows acanthosis, elongation of the rete ridges, hyperkeratosis. The dermal infiltrate has decreased and is in close approximation only around one hair follicle. (× 13)

FIG. 6-16

Lichen planus, hypertrophic form, higher magnification of Fig. 6-15. The lower part of the hair follicle is surrounded by a dense chronic inflammatory infiltrate. The basal cells are destroyed. (× 40)

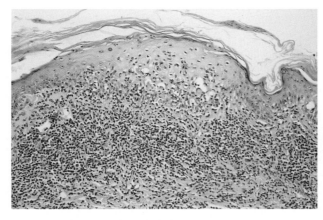

FIG. 6-17

Benign lichenoid keratosis. Within the epidermis several Civatte bodies can be seen. A dense, bandlike subepidermal infiltrate is seen that presses against the epidermis. Except for the absence of hypergranulosis, there is considerable resemblance to lichen planus. (× 40)

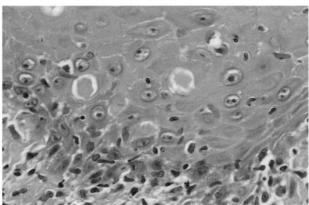

FIG. 6-18

Benign lichenoid keratosis. In the lower epidermis colloid bodies or Civatte bodies can be seen. They have a homogenous, eosinophilic appearance. They represent degenerated keratinocytes. (× 240)

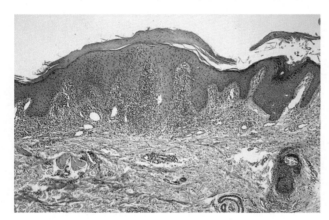

FIG. 6-19

Keratosis lichenoides chronica. The epidermis shows parakeratosis. There is a dense, lymphocytic subepidermal infiltrate that is bandlike, as in lichen planus. (× 16)

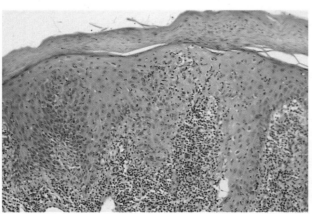

FIG. 6-20

Keratosis lichenoides chronica. Except for the parakeratosis and absence of a granular layer, the histologic picture greatly resembles lichen planus. (× 40)

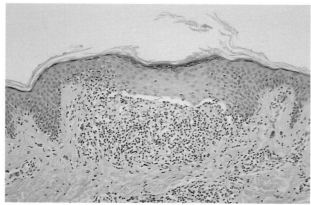

FIG. 6-21

Lichen nitidus. A circumscribed infiltrate is closely attached to the lower surface of the epidermis. The basal layer is absent, and the epidermis is partially detached from the dermis. (× 40)

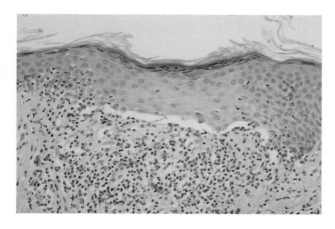

FIG. 6-22

Lichen nitidus, higher magnification of Fig. 6-21. Most of the cells within the infiltrate are lymphocytes and macrophages. Several of the macrophages have the appearance of epithelioid cells. (× 64)

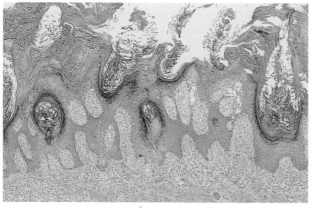

FIG. 6-23

Inflammatory linear verrucous epidermal nevus. The epidermis shows hyperkeratosis with foci of parakeratosis, moderate acanthosis, and elongation of the rete ridges. (× 13)

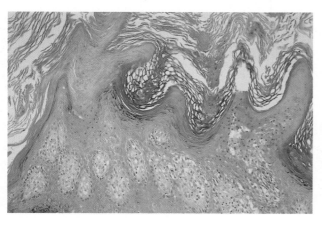

FIG. 6-24

Inflammatory linear verrucous epidermal nevus. A characteristic feature is seen, consisting of a regular alternation of parakeratotic areas without a granular layer and slightly depressed, hyperkeratotic areas with a distinct granular layer. (× 40)

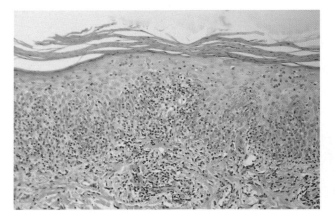

FIG. 6-25

Pityriasis lichenoides et varioliformis acuta.
There is marked exocytosis of lymphoid cells and extravasation of erythrocytes. ($\times$ 40)

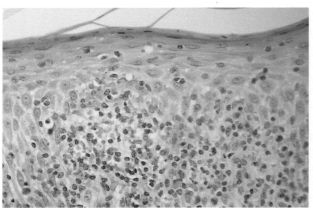

FIG. 6-26

Pityriasis lichenoides et varioliformis acuta.
A pronounced mononuclear infiltrate is present in the dermis and is seen invading the epidermis. Erythrocytes are trapped within the epidermis, which is a characteristic feature of the disease. ($\times$ 64)

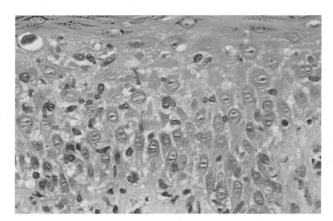

FIG. 6-27

Pityriasis lichenoides et varioliformis acuta.
The epidermis shows spongiosis and "trapped" erythrocytes. ($\times$ 160)

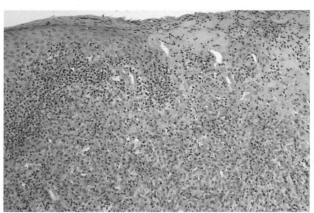

FIG. 6-28

Pityriasis lichenodes et varioliformis acuta.
There is a dense inflammatory infiltrate of mononuclear cells in the upper dermis with invasion into the epidermis. On the right side the epidermis has become necrotic. ($\times$ 40)

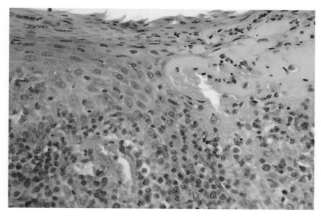

FIG. 6-29

Pityriasis lichenoides et varioliformis acuta, higher magnification of Fig. 6-28. The epidermis is necrotic on the right side. A dense, lymphocytic infiltrate is present beneath the epidermis, with exocytosis into the epidermis. Erythrocytes are trapped within the necrotic and the intact epidermis. (× 64)

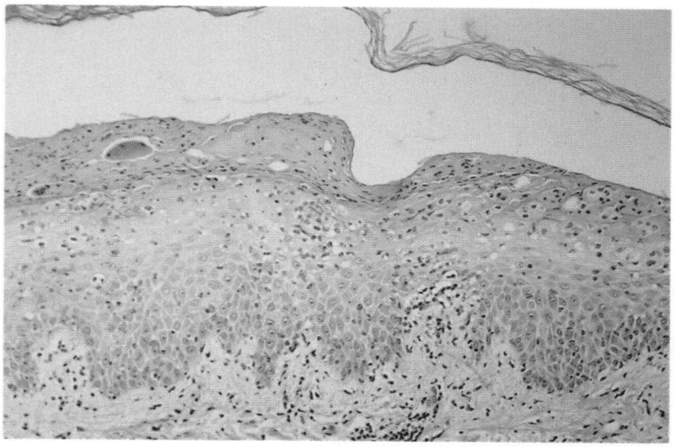

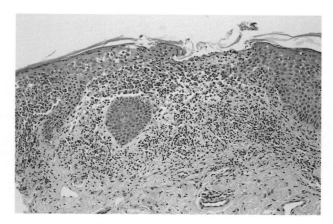

FIG. 6-30

Pityriasis lichenoides et varioliformis acuta. The epidermis has become necrotic and stains eosinophilic in its upper portion. The non-necrotic epidermis beneath stains only weakly with H&E. (× 40)

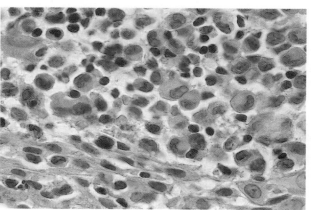

FIG. 6-31

Lymphomatoid papulosis. The infiltrate contains many cells with an atypical appearance. Two types of atypical-appearing cells occur, referred to as type A and type B. In this illustration cells of type A predominate: large rounded cells with vesicular nuclei and abundant cytoplasm. (× 64)

FIG. 6-32

Lymphomatoid papulosis, higher magnification of Fig. 6-31. Some of the large atypical-appearing type A cells are multinucleated. They resemble the Reed-Sternberg cells seen in Hodgkin's disease. (× 240)

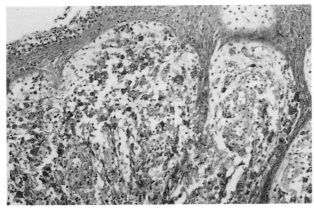

FIG. 6-33

Lymphomatoid papulosis. Giemsa stain. The infiltrate shows many atypical-appearing cells. In this illustration type B cells predominate, which have large, irregularly shaped hyperchromatic nuclei. (× 64)

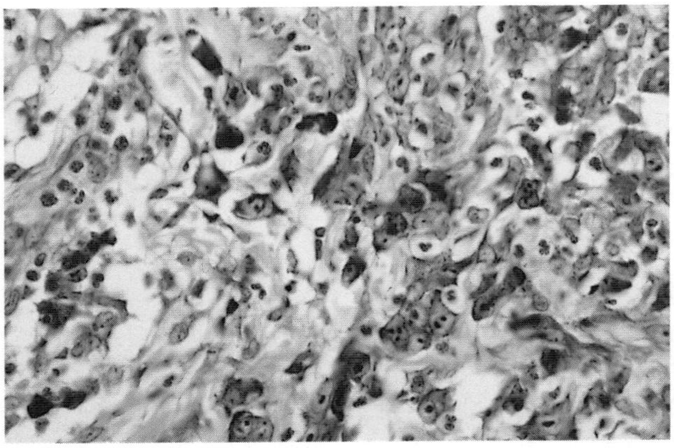

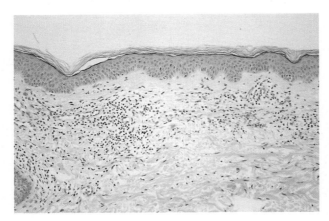

FIG. 6-34

Lymphomatoid papulosis, higher magnification of Fig. 6-33. Many of the irregularly shaped, hyperchromatic nuclei resemble mycosis cells, as seen in mycosis fungoides. (× 160)

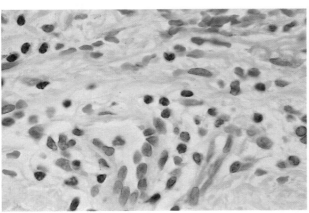

FIG. 6-35

Purpura pigmentosa chronica. The epidermis looks normal. A perivascular cellular infiltrate consisting of lymphocytes and macrophages can be seen in the upper dermis. Small amounts of extravasated red cells are present. (× 40)

FIG. 6-36

Purpura pigmentosa chronica, higher magnification of Fig. 6-25. Within the infiltrate of lymphocytes and macrophages extravasated erythrocytes can be seen. (× 240)

CHAPTER 7

Vascular
Diseases

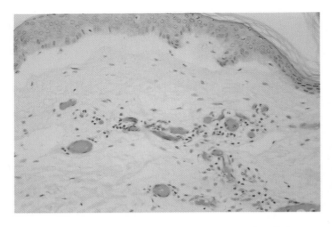

FIG. 7-1

Coumarin necrosis. The capillaries in the upper part of the dermis are occluded with fibrin and platelet thrombi. There are no signs of inflammation of the blood vessels. (× 64)

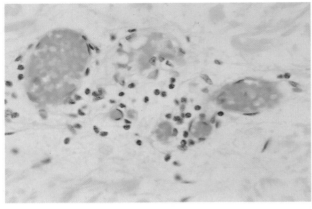

FIG. 7-2

Coumarin necrosis, higher magnification. The capillaries are occluded with fibrin and platelet thrombi. (× 240)

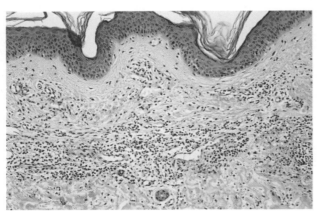

FIG. 7-3

Leukocytoclastic vasculitis. The epidermis looks normal. A perivascular infiltrate is present predominantly consisting of neutrophils. (× 40)

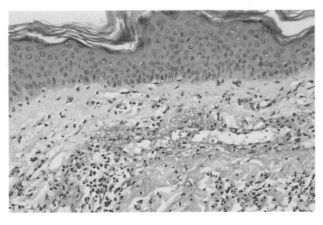

FIG. 7-4

Leukocytoclastic vasculitis. A cellular infiltrate has invaded the vessel wall. The outline of the blood vessel is indistinct owing to deposition of fibrinoid material around them. The infiltrate consists of neutrophils and mononuclear cells. (× 64)

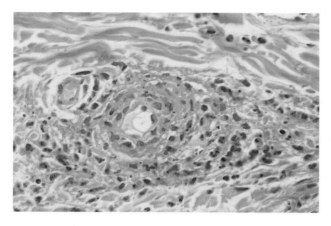

FIG. 7-5

Leukocytoclastic vasculitis. The endothelial cells are swollen; the vessel wall is infiltrated by inflammatory cells; fibrinoid material is deposited within and around the vessel wall. The infiltrate is largely composed of neutrophils, many of which show fragmentation of their nuclei. (× 160)

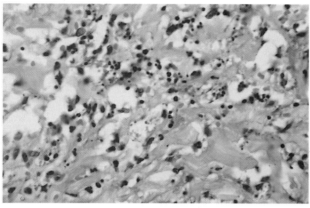

FIG. 7-6

Leukocytoclastic vasculitis. The cellular infiltrate consists of neutrophils, many of which show fragmentation of their nuclei. There is extravasation of erythrocytes. (× 160)

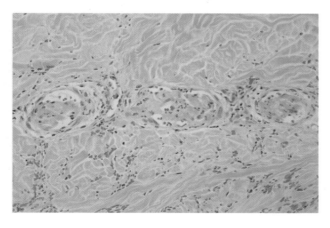

FIG. 7-7

Monoclonal cryoglobulinemia. The capillaries are filled with an amorphous eosinophilic material. Extensive extravasation of erythrocytes is present. (× 64)

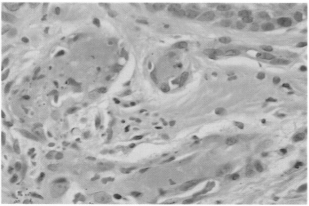

FIG. 7-8

Monoclonal cryoglobulinemia. The capillaries are occluded with an eosinophilic amorphous material consisting of precipitated cryoglobulin. (× 160)

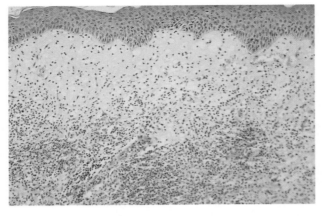

FIG. 7-9

Acute febrile neutrophilic dermatosis (Sweet's syndrome). The upper dermis shows edema. In the lower dermis a dense perivascular infiltrate can be seen. (× 40)

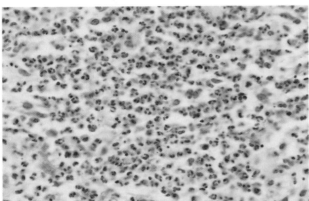

FIG. 7-10

Acute febrile neutrophilic dermatosis (Sweet's syndrome). The infiltrate mainly consists of neutrophils with a few mononuclear cells mixed in. (× 160)

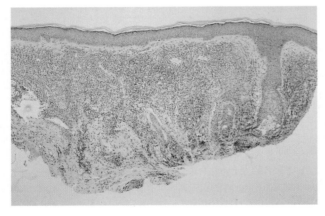

FIG. 7-11

Granuloma faciale. A dense polymorphous infiltrate is found. The infiltrate does not invade the epidermis or the pilosebaceous appendages, but is separated from them by a narrow grenz zone of normal collagen. (× 16)

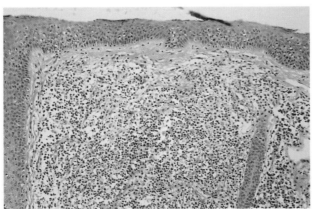

FIG. 7-12

Granuloma faciale. The dense polymorphous infiltrate is separated from the epidermis by a narrow grenz zone of normal collagen. The infiltrate contains many eosinophils. (× 40)

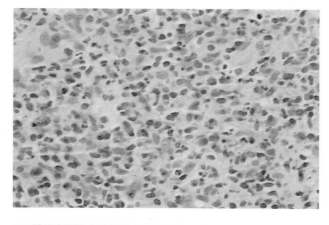

FIG. 7·13

Granuloma faciale. The infiltrate consists of eosinophils, neutrophils, and mononuclear cells. (× 160)

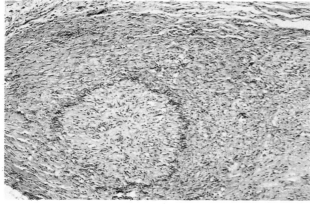

FIG. 7·14

Temporal giant cell arteritis, Verhoeff elastic tissue stain. The lumen of the artery is occluded, and there is damage to the internal elastic lamina on the left side. (× 40)

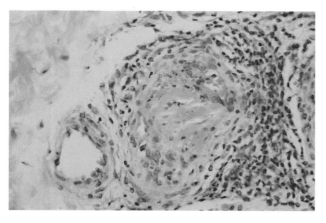

FIG. 7·15

Atrophie blanche. A dermal vessel shows almost complete occlusion by eosinophilic fibrinoid material. A dense perivascular infiltrate consisting of mononuclear cells can be seen. (× 160)

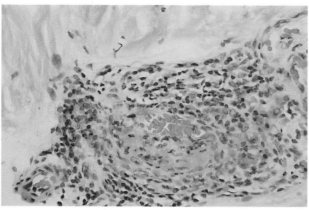

FIG. 7·16

Atrophie blanche. The capillary contains eosinophilic material in a portion of its wall. There is a dense perivascular infiltrate consisting of mononuclear cells. (× 160)

CHAPTER 8

Inflammatory Diseases of the Epidermal Appendages and of Cartilage

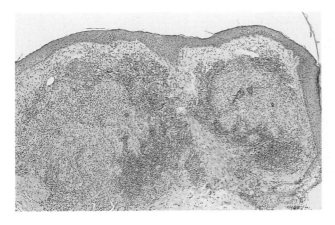

FIG. 8-1

Acne rosacea. In the papular type of the disease a granulomatous infiltrate can be seen. The islands are composed of epithelioid cells and a few giant cells, and are surrounded by lymphocytes, resulting in a tuberculoid picture. (× 13)

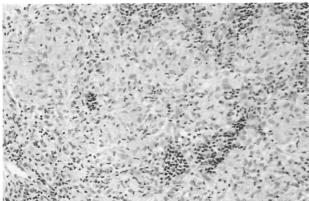

FIG. 8-2

Acne rosacea, papular type, higher magnification of Fig. 8-1. The tuberculoid infiltrate consisting of epithelioid cells in the center and lymphocytes at the periphery is evident. There is no central necrosis. (× 40)

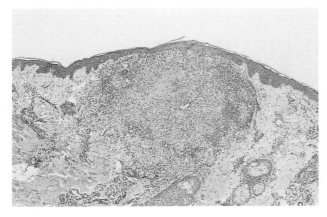

FIG. 8-3

Lupus miliaris disseminatus faciei. A "tubercle" is seen in the dermis. In the center of the tubercle caseation necrosis is seen, which is surrounded by epithelioid cells and lymphocytes. (× 13)

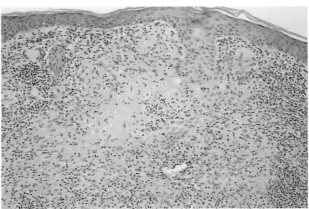

FIG. 8-4

Lupus miliaris disseminatus faciei. In the center of the "tubercle" amorphous caseation necrosis is seen, surrounded by epithelioid cells. At the periphery of the tubercle a chronic inflammatory infiltrate is seen. (× 40)

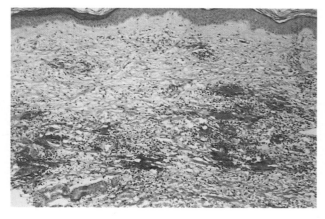

FIG. 8-5

Eosinophilic cellulitis (Wells' syndrome). In the dermis elongated areas of homogeneous eosinophilic material are seen. They are surrounded by eosinophils and macrophages. These elongated areas are referred to as flame figures. (Courtesy of R. K. Winkelman, M.D.) (× 40)

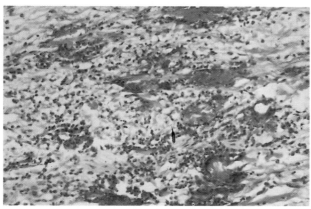

FIG. 8-6

Eosinophilic cellulitis (Wells' syndrome). The flame figures form secondary to the disintegration of eosinophils and consist of aggregates of eosinophilic granules and nuclear fragments coating intact collagen fibers. (Courtesy of R. K. Winkelman, M.D.) (× 64)

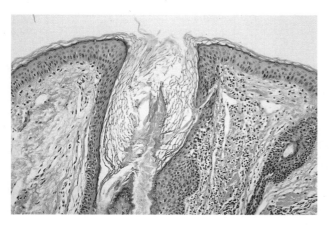

FIG. 8-7

Infundibulofolliculitis. The uppermost portion of the hair follicle (infundibulum) is dilated and shows spongiosis at its wall. The surrounding dermis shows a mild chronic inflammatory infiltrate. (× 40)

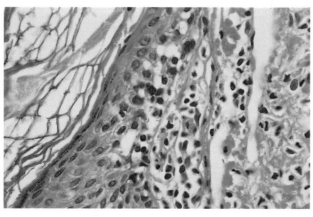

FIG. 8-8

Infundibulofolliculitis. There is spongiosis of the wall of the infundibulum. Exocytosis of inflammatory cells from the dermis into the spongiotic areas is usually seen. (× 160)

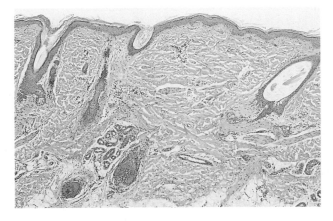

FIG. 8-9

Alopecia areata. The characteristic finding is the presence of miniature hair structures. The miniature telogen hair structure on the left is surrounded by a thick fibrous root sheath. (× 13)

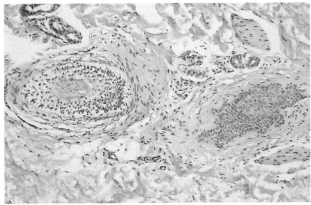

FIG. 8-10

Alopecia areata. Both hair follicles are surrounded by a thick fibrous wall. The miniature hair structure is surrounded by a mild lymphocytic infiltrate. (× 40)

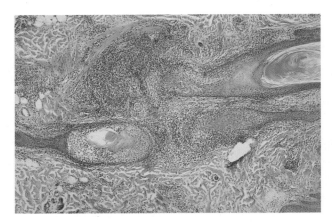

FIG. 8-11

Alopecia mucinosa, H&E stain. There is a dense mononuclear infiltrate around the hair follicles. The hair follicles show mucinous changes; the hair follicle on the left shows a cystic space. (× 16)

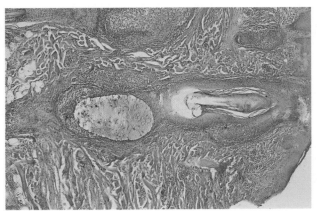

FIG. 8-12

Alopecia mucinosa, alcian stain. The cystic space in the hair follicle contains mucin, which stains blue with alcian. (× 16)

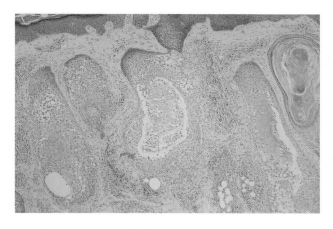

FIG. 8-13

Alopecia mucinosa. Several pilosebaceous follicles show "reticular" degeneration of its cells associated with mucin. (× 16)

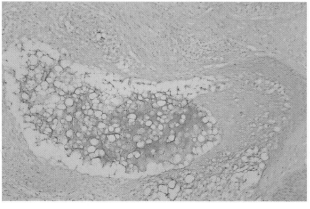

FIG. 8-14

Alopecia mucinosa, alcian stain. The cystic space is filled with mucin, which stains blue. (× 64)

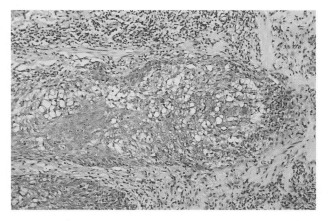

FIG. 8-15

Alopecia mucinosa. The mucinous material stains metachromatically with toluidine blue. (× 40)

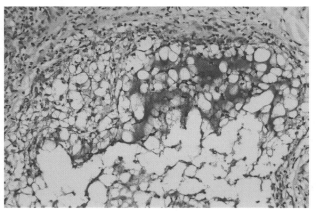

FIG. 8-16

Alopecia mucinosa. A cystic space has formed within the outer root sheath. It is filled with mucin, which stains metachromatically with toluidine blue. (× 64)

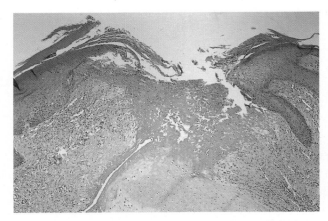

FIG. 8-17

Chondrodermatitis nodulars helicis. The epidermis shows an ulcer. The base of the ulcer is formed by degenerated collagen, which shows richly vascularized granulation tissue on both sides. (× 16)

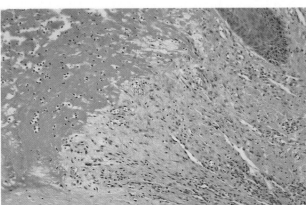

FIG. 8-18

Chondrodermatitis nodularis helicis, higher magnification of Fig. 8-17. The base of the ulcer is seen. Through the ulcer necrotic dermal debris is being eliminated. The necrotic material is surrounded by richly vascularized granulation tissue. (× 40)

CHAPTER 9

Inflammatory Diseases Due to Physical Agents and Foreign Substances

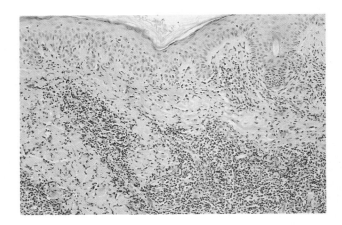

FIG. 9-1

Polymorhous light eruption, plaque type. In the dermis a patchy lymphocytic infiltrate can be seen, as in lupus erythematosus. However, there is no hydropic degeneration of the basal cells. (× 40)

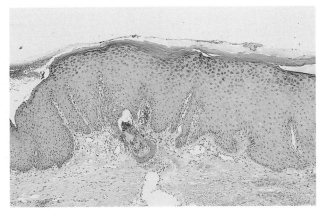

FIG. 9-2

Radiation dermatitis, late stage. The epidermis is hyperplastic and shows a downward growth around a telangiectatic blood vessel. (× 13)

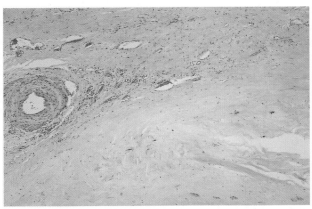

FIG. 9-3

Radiation dermatitis, late stage. The collagen bundles in the lower half of the picture are hyalinized and appear faintly eosinophilic. (× 16)

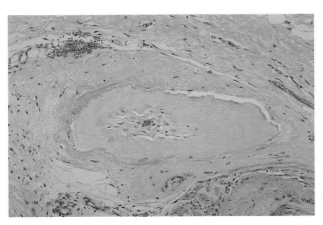

FIG. 9-4

Radiation dermatitis, late stage. The blood vessel is thrombosed and shows recanalization. The surrounding collagen is hyalinized. (× 40)

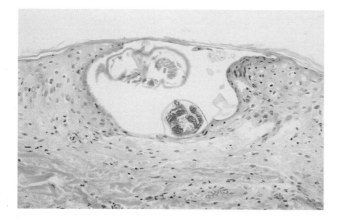

FIG. 9-5

Scabies. A burrow is located in the stratum corneum. A female mite is located in the burrow. (× 64)

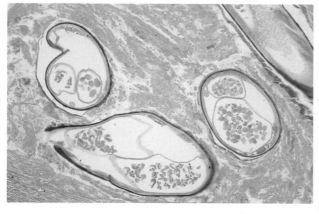

FIG. 9-6

Onchocerciasis. Transverse and diagonal sections of the adult filaria *Onchocerca* are located in the dermis. They are surrounded by dense fibrous tissue. (× 40)

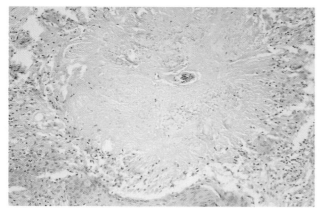

FIG. 9-7

Schistosomiasis. An ovum is seen within an area of necrosis. The necrotic tissue is surrounded by a palisading granuloma. (× 40)

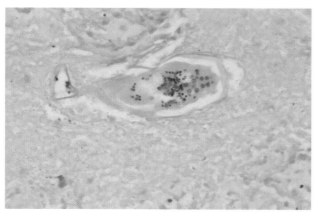

FIG. 9-8

Schistosomiasis, higher magnification of Fig. 9-7. The ovum of *Schistosoma mansoni* shows a spine on its lateral aspect. (× 160)

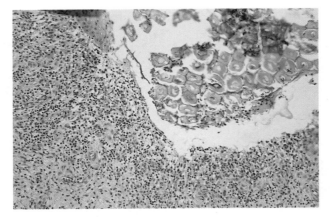

FIG. 9-9

Foreign body reaction caused by fragments of a plant. They are surrounded by a chronic infiltrate consisting of giant cells, lymphocytes, and macrophages. (× 40)

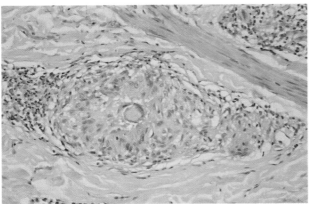

FIG. 9-10

Foreign body granuloma owing to suture material. The granuloma consists of epithelioid cells and foreign body giant cells. At the periphery of the granuloma, lymphocytes can be seen. (× 64)

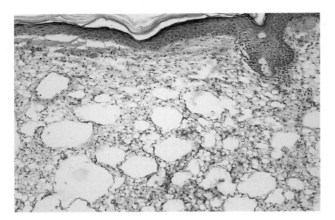

FIG. 9-11

Silicone granuloma. The ovoid or round cavities represent spaces filled with vegetable oil. Silicone gels contain vegetable oils, fatty acids, and silicone. (× 40)

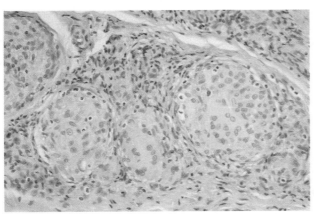

FIG. 9-12

Silica granuloma. Epithelioid cell tubercles are present that contain multinucleated giant cells but only a few lymphoid cells. (× 64)

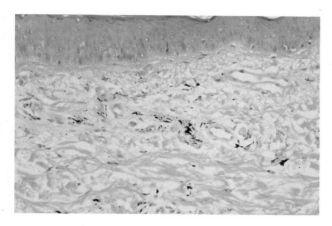

FIG. 9-13

Tattoo. Diffusely scattered granules of dye can be seen extracellularly in the corium without any inflammatory reaction. (× 40)

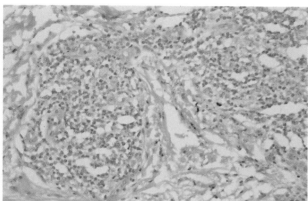

FIG. 9-14

Tattoo granuloma. Epithelioid cell granulomas can be seen, as in sarcoidosis. A few tattoo granules can still be seen between both granulomas. (× 64)

CHAPTER 10

Noninfectious Granulomas

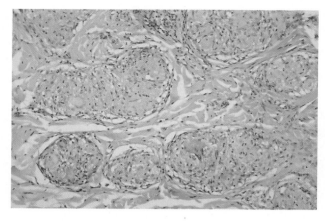

FIG. 10-1

Sarcoidosis. Circumscribed granulomas of epithelioid cells showing little or no central necrosis can be seen. At the periphery of each granuloma a few scattered lymphocytes can be seen. Several foreign body giant cells are present. (× 40)

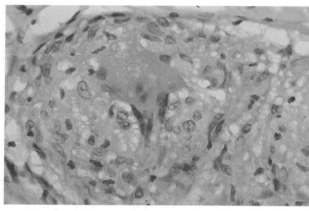

FIG. 10-2

Sarcoidosis, higher magnification of Fig. 10-1. An epithelioid granuloma with a central large giant cell can be seen. (× 240)

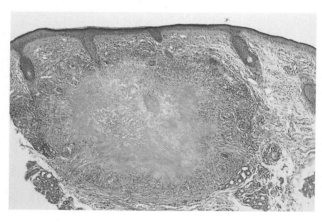

FIG. 10-3

Granuloma annulare. A focus of complete collagen degeneration is seen, surrounded by marcophages in a palisading or radial arrangement. At the periphery of the granuloma, lymphocytes can be seen. (× 16)

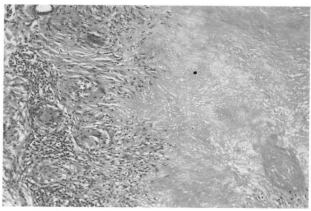

FIG. 10-4

Granuloma annulare, higher magnification of the edge of the granuloma. The radial arrangement of the macrophages can be seen. The collagen shows complete degeneration. (× 40)

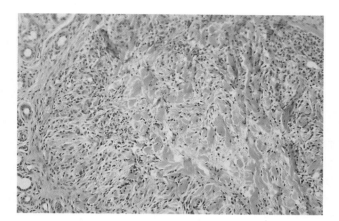

FIG. 10-5

Granuloma annulare, incomplete collagen degeneration. Foci of incomplete degeneration consist of ill-defined areas in which some of the collagen bundles appear normal, whereas others are found in various stages of degeneration ranging from a slight decrease in eosinophilic staining to replacement by mucinous material. (× 40)

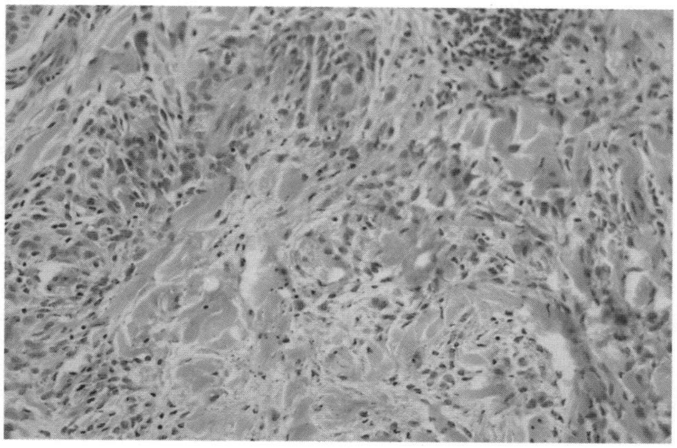

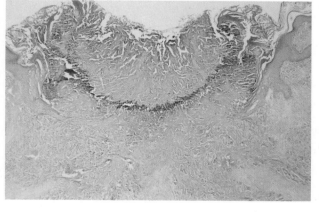

FIG. 10-6

Granuloma annulare. Ill-defined areas of incomplete collagen degeneration have been replaced by mucinous material. (× 64)

FIG. 10-7

Perforating granuloma annulare. A focus of complete collagen degeneration surrounded by a wall of inflammatory cells is located within an ulcerated area of the epidermis. (× 10)

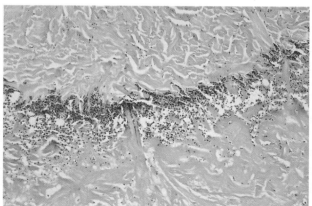

FIG. 10-8

Perforating granuloma annulare, higher magnification of Fig. 10-7. The perforated material consists of completely degenerated collagen, which is surrounded by palisading histiocytes. (× 160)

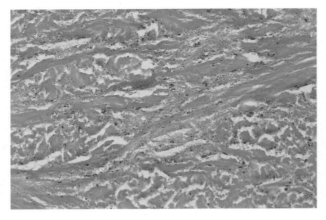

FIG. 10-9

Necrobiosis lipoidica, necrobiotic type. Poorly defined areas of granular basophilic necrobiotic collagen are seen intermingled with almost normal collagen. The collagen bundles are split up, amorphous and anuclear. (× 64)

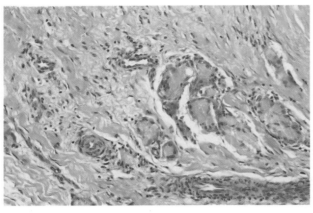

FIG. 10-10

Necrobiosis lipoidica. Scattered foreign body giant cells are frequently present in necrobiosis lipoidica and are of considerable value. (× 64)

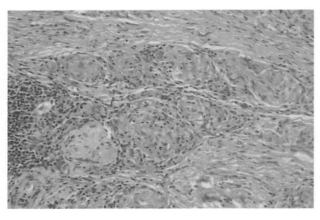

FIG. 10-11

Necrobiosis lipoidica. In the granulomatous type of reaction the dermis contains scattered granulomas consisting of epithelioid cells, macrophages, giant cells, and lymphocytes. (× 64)

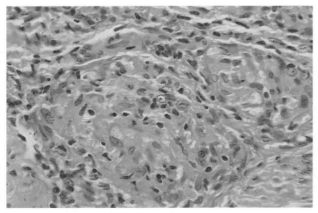

FIG. 10-12

Necrobiosis lipoidica. Higher magnification of a granuloma composed of epithelioid cells, lymphocytes, and macrophages. (× 160)

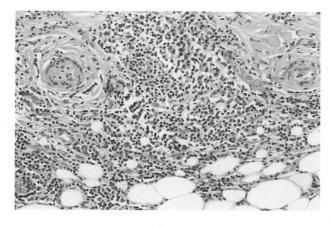

FIG. 10-13

Necrobiosis lipoidica. The blood vessels in the lower dermis show proliferation of their endothelial cells, which has led to partial occlusion of the lumen. (× 40)

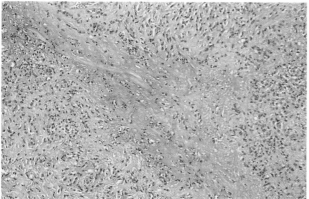

FIG. 10-14

Rheumatoid nodule. There is a sharply demarcated focus of fibrinoid collagen degeneration surrounded by macrophages. The lesion is located in the subcutaneous tissue. (× 40)

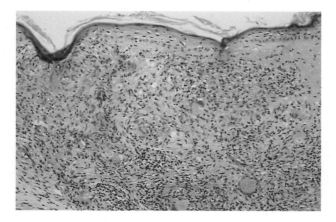

FIG. 10-15

Annular elastolytic granuloma. Numerous large giant cells can be seen. Several of them contain asteroid bodies. In addition, there is an infiltrate of epithelioid cells, macrophages, and lymphocytes. (× 40)

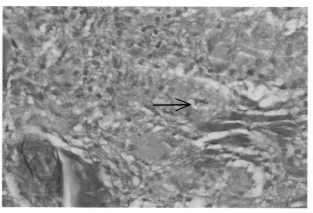

FIG. 10-16

Annular elastolytic granuloma, elastic tissue stain. Within the area of an accumulation of giant cells, most, if not all, elastic fibers have been destroyed. The asteroid body within the giant cell stains like elastic fibers (arrow). (× 160)

CHAPTER 11

Inflammatory Diseases of the Subcutaneous Fat

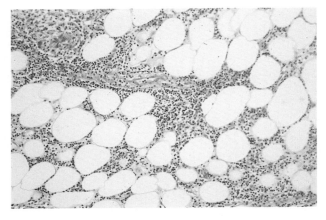

FIG. 11-1

Erythema nodosum. A chronic inflammatory infiltrate has extended from an interlobular septum into a fat lobule in a lacelike fashion. The infiltrate consists of lymphocytes, macrophages, and neutrophils. (× 40)

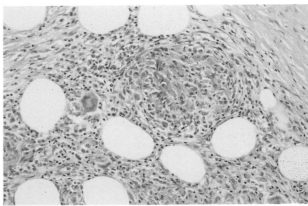

FIG. 11-2

Erythema nodosum. A giant cell can be seen as well as an occluded blood vessel. The vessel wall is infiltrated with mononuclear inflammatory cells. (× 64)

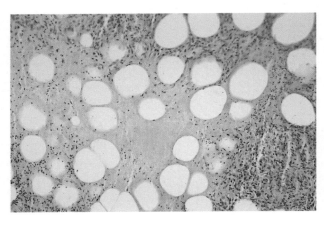

FIG. 11-3

Erythema induratum. Within the subcutaneous fat an area of caseation necrosis can be seen. A mononuclear infiltrate extends between the fat cells, which are still quite well preserved. (× 40)

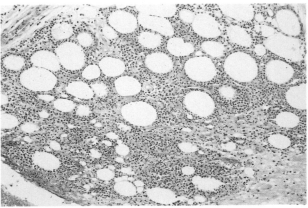

FIG. 11-4

Relapsing febrile nodular nonsuppurative panniculitis (Weber-Christian disease), first stage. An acute inflammatory infiltrate predominantly consisting of neutrophils extends between the fat cells. (× 40)

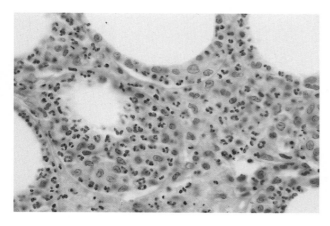

FIG. 11-5

Relapsing febrile nodular nonsuppurative panniculitis (Weber-Christian disease), first stage. The inflammatory infiltrate predominantly consists of neutrophils with an admixture of macrophages. (× 160)

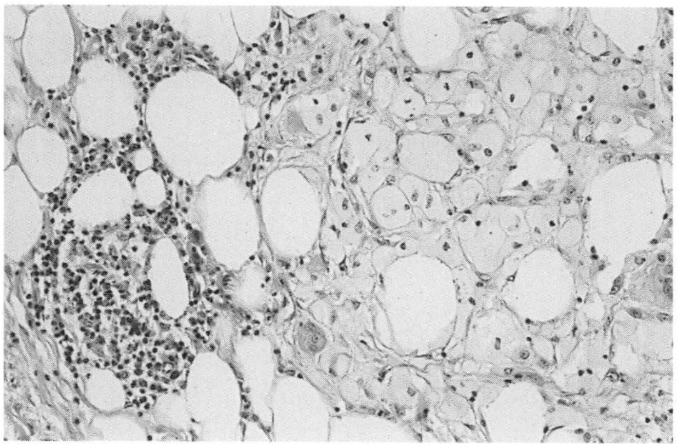

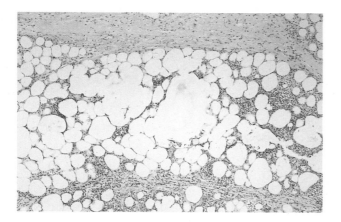

FIG. 11-6

Relapsing febrile nodular nonsuppurative panniculitis (Weber-Christian disease), second stage. Macrophages have started to digest fat cells and have become foam cells. (× 64)

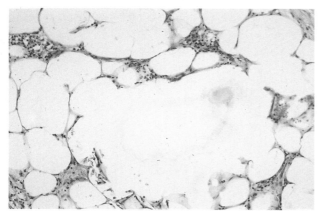

FIG. 11-7

Cold panniculitis. Some of the fat cells in the subcutaneous fat have ruptured. They are surrounded by an inflammatory infiltrate consisting of neutrophils, lymphocytes, macrophages, and a few eosinophils. (× 16)

FIG. 11-8

Cold panniculitis, higher magnification. Fat cells have ruptured and coalesced to form cystic spaces. (× 40)

CHAPTER 12

Eruptions Due to Drugs

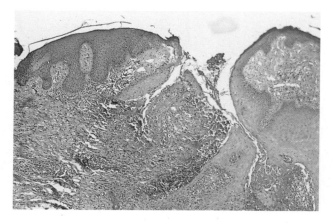

FIG. 12-1

Penicillamine-induced elastosis perforans serpiginosa. There is a narrow transepidermal channel. The base of the channel shows necrobiotic material consisting of degenerated inflammatory cells and degenerated elastic fibers. (× 16)

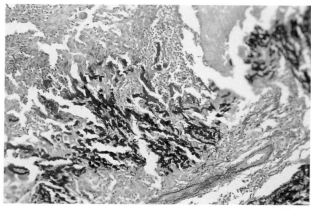

FIG. 12-2

Penicillamine-induced elastosis perforans serpiginosa, elastic tissue stain. The base of the transepidermal channel consists of necrotic inflammatory cells and elastic fibers. (× 40)

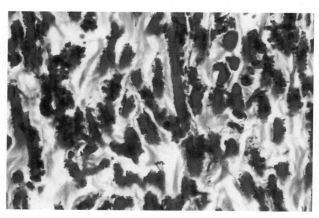

FIG. 12-3

Penicillamine-induced elastosis perforans serpiginosa, elastic tissue stain. The elastic fibers are hyperplastic and have an appearance that is specific for this disease: they show lateral budding with the buds arranged perpendicular to the principal fibers. These elastic fibers have been compared to the twigs of a bramble bush. (× 160)

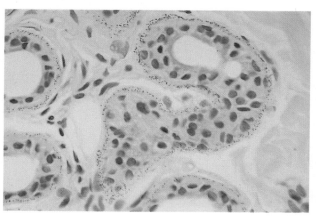

FIG. 12-4

Argyria. Silver granules are found in the membrana propria of the sweat glands. (× 160)

CHAPTER 13

Degenerative
Diseases

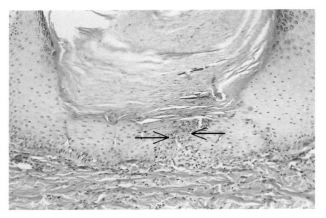

FIG. 13-1

Kyrle's disease. The epidermis shows an invagination that is filled with a parakeratotic plug containing basophilic debris. The base of the invagination shows a narrow channel (arrows) through which the plug is in direct contact with the dermis. The invagination shows a well-developed granular layer except at the points at which the parakeratotic cells of the plug are in direct contact with the epidermis. (× 64)

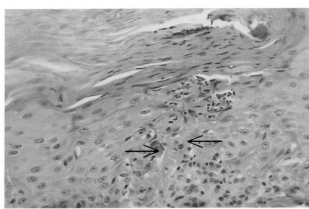

FIG. 13-2

Kyrle's disease, higher magnification of Fig. 13-1. There is a disruption of the epidermal cells. Thus the plug is in direct contact with the dermis, which, in this area, shows degeneration with inflammatory cells. (× 160)

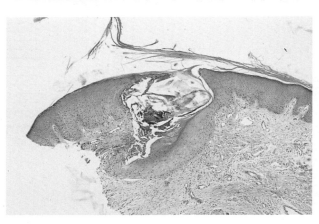

FIG. 13-3

Perforating folliculitis. Within a dilated hair follicle, orthokeratotic and parakeratotic material is seen that is intermingled with basophilic debris. (× 16)

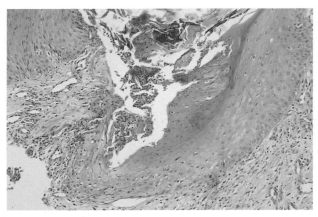

FIG. 13-4

Perforating folliculitis, higher magnification of Fig. 13-3. Within a dilated hair follicle a perforation of the follicular epithelium can be seen. At the site of perforation the dermis shows an inflammatory infiltrate containing degenerated collagen. (× 40)

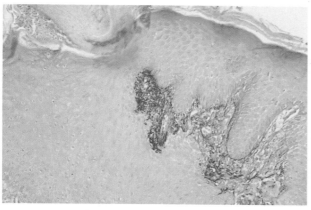

FIG. 13-5

Elastosis perforans serpiginosa, elastic tissue stain. A transepidermal channel can be seen through which elastic fibers are eliminated. The elastic fibers in the upper corium and in the papillae are increased in number. The epidermis is hyperplastic. ($\times$ 40)

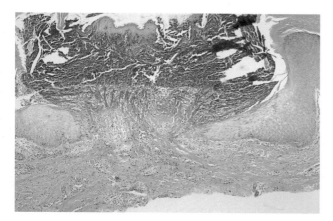

FIG. 13-6

Elastosis perforans serpiginosa, elastic tissue stain, higher magnification of Fig. 13-5. The transepidermal channel is filled with elastic fibers. ($\times$ 160)

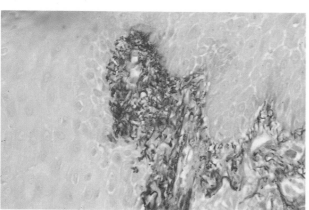

FIG. 13-7

Reactive perforating collagenosis. The epidermis has formed a cup-shaped depression that contains basophilic collagen and numerous pyknotic nuclei of inflammatory cells. The epidermis is perforated. Through this perforation the basophilic collagen is being extruded into the cup-shaped invagination. ($\times$ 16)

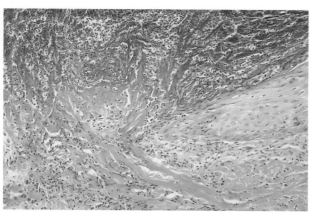

FIG. 13-8

Reactive perforating collagenosis, higher magnification of Fig. 13-7 showing the area of perforation and extrusion of vertically arranged collagen from the dermis into the cup-shaped invagination. ($\times$ 40)

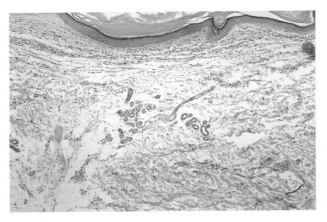

FIG. 13-9

Acrodermatitis chronica atrophicans. The epidermis is atrophic, and the hair and sebaceous glands have disappeared. Because of the atrophy of the dermis, the sweat glands lie unusually close to the epidermis. (× 16)

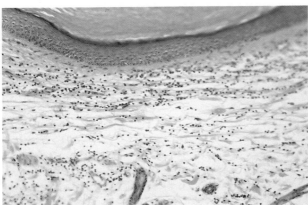

FIG. 13-10

Acrodermatitis chronica atrophicans, higher magnification of Fig. 13-9. Under an atrophic epidermis a narrow zone of normal collagen can be seen. Underneath this grenz zone a bandlike infiltrate of mononuclear cells can be seen. The dermis shows interstitial edema and atrophy of the collagen bundles. (× 64)

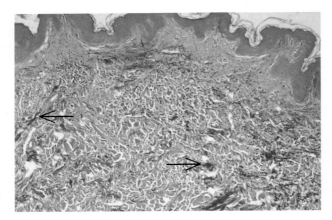

FIG. 13-11

Macular atrophy (anetoderma), elastic tissue stain. In the center of the micrograph the elastic fibers have disappeared; on the right and left sides they are decreased in number (arrows). (× 16)

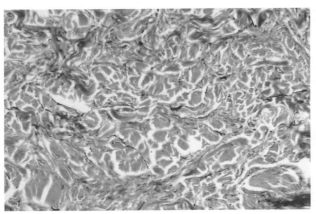

FIG. 13-12

Macular atrophy (anetoderma), elastic tissue stain, higher magnification of Fig. 13-11. In the upper left corner of the micrograph the elastic fibers are greatly reduced in number. (× 40)

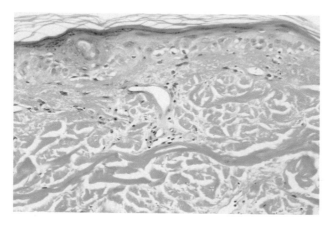

FIG. 13-13

Lichen sclerosus et atrophicus. This early lesion shows atrophy of the epidermis with hydropic degeneration of the basal cells. The dermis shows edema. (× 40)

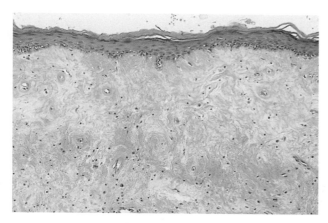

FIG. 13-14

Lichen sclerosus et atrophicus. The stratum malpighii is atrophic, and there is marked lymphedema of the upper dermis. A diffuse mononuclear inflammatory infiltrate can be seen in the middermis. (× 40)

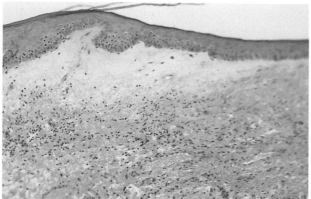

FIG. 13-15

Lichen sclerosus et atrophicus. Beneath the atrophic epidermis a broad zone of lymphedema can be seen. Within this zone the collagenous fibers are swollen and homogeneous. They stain poorly with eosin. The blood and lymph vessels are dilated. (× 40)

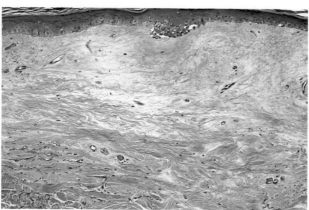

FIG. 13-16

Lichen sclerosus et atrophicus, elastic tissue stain, late lesion. The elastic fibers are absent within the area of lymphedema. (× 40)

CHAPTER 14

Bacterial
Diseases

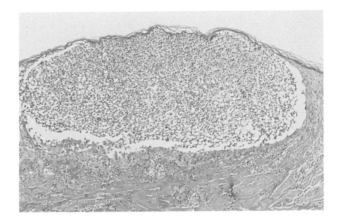

FIG. 14-1

Impetigo. A large pustule underneath the stratum corneum can be seen. It contains numerous neutrophils. (× 16)

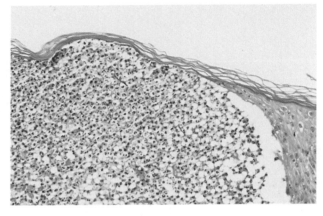

FIG. 14-2

Impetigo, higher magnification of Fig. 14-1. The pustule has arisen within the granular layer and is filled with neutrophils and nuclear debris. (× 40)

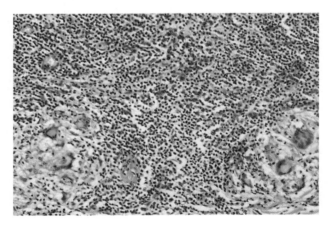

FIG. 14-3

Tuberculosis, lupus vulgaris. In the upper dermis several tubercles composed of epithelioid cells and foreign body giant cells are present. A dense infiltrate of macrophages and lymphocytes can be seen between the tubercles. (× 16)

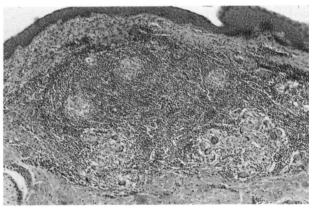

FIG. 14-4

Tuberculosis, lupus vulgaris, higher magnification of Fig. 14-3. Small tubercles of epithelioid cells and giant cells (Langhans type) can be seen intermingled with a dense infiltrate of predominantly lymphocytes. (× 40)

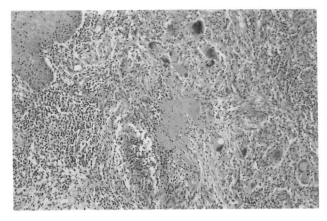

FIG. 14-5

Swimming pool granuloma caused by *Mycobacterium marinum*. In the center of a granuloma an area of necrosis can be seen, which is surrounded by multinucleated foreign body giant cells, macrophages, and lymphocytes. (× 40)

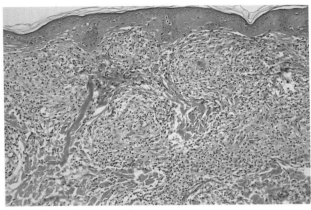

FIG. 14-6

Tuberculoid leprosy. Several epithelioid cell granulomas can be seen in the dermis that are indistinguishable from those seen in sarcoidosis. At the periphery of the granumolas an admixture of lymphocytes can be seen. (× 40)

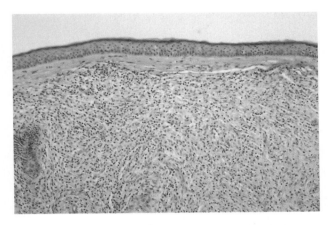

FIG. 14-7

Lepromatous leprosy. There is an extensive cellular infiltrate in the dermis that is separated from the epidermis by a narrow grenz zone of normal collagen. Macrophages predominate. The infiltrate causes the destruction of cutaneous appendages. (× 40)

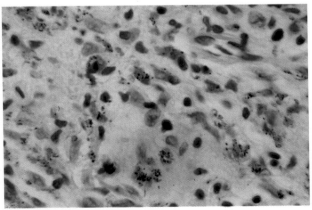

FIG. 14-8

Lepromatous leprosy, Fite stain. Numerous acid-fast red-staining lepra bacilli are seen within lepra cells or Virchow cells. (× 240)

CHAPTER 15

Treponemal Diseases

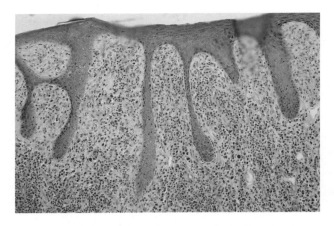

FIG. 15-1

Primary syphilis. The epidermis shows slight acanthosis with an elongation of the rete ridges. A dense infiltrate composed of lymphocytes and many plasma cells is present in the dermis. (× 40)

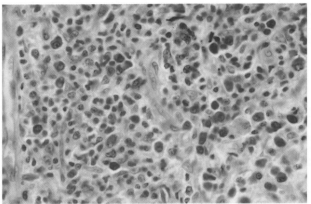

FIG. 15-2

Primary syphilis, higher magnification. The inflammatory infiltrate consists of lymphocytes and plasma cells. (× 160)

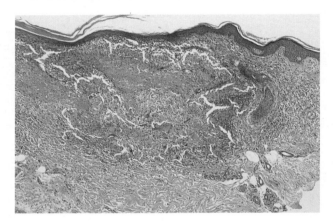

FIG. 15-3

Tertiary syphilis. This gumma shows extensive caseation necrosis in the dermis. Epithelioid cells and giant cells are present. (× 16)

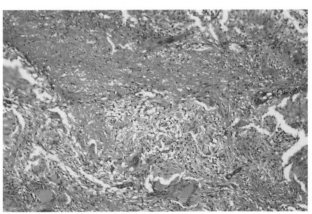

FIG. 15-4

Tertiary syphilis, higher magnification of Fig. 15-3. The large area of caseation necrosis is surrounded by several multinucleated giant cells. (× 40)

CHAPTER 16

Fungal
Diseases

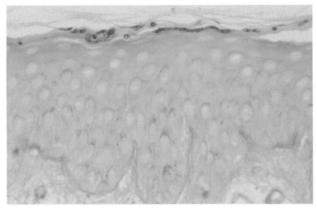

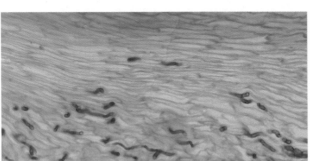

FIG. 16-1

Tinea versicolor, periodic acid-Schiff stain (PAS). The horny layer contains hyphae and spores, often referred to as spaghetti and meatballs. (× 160)

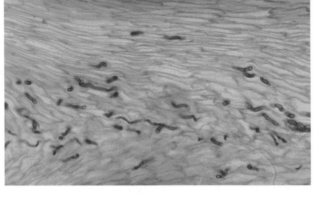

FIG. 16-2

Onychomycosis, PAS stain. Hyphae can be seen within the stratum corneum of a toe nail. (× 160)

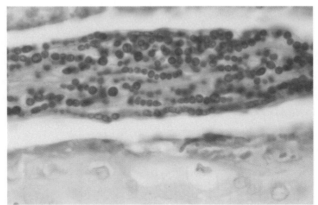

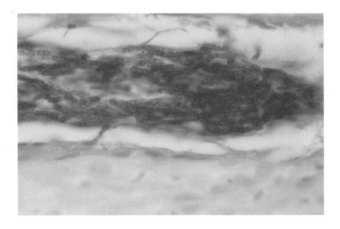

FIG. 16-3 and FIG. 16-4

Trichophyton rubrum within a hair. The fungus can be present either as spores (Fig. 16-3) or as hyphae (Fig. 16-4). (× 240)

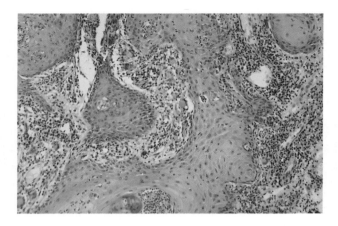

FIG. 16-5

North American blastomycosis. The epidermis shows hyperplasia. A dense inflammatory infiltrate containing multinucleated giant cells can be seen in the dermis. (× 40)

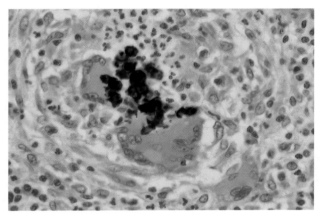

FIG. 16-6

North American blastomycosis. The spores of *Blastomyces dermatitidis* are seen either within giant cells or lying free in the tissue. The spores have a thick wall that gives them a double-contoured appearance. The extracellular spores are surrounded by numerous neutrophils. (× 160)

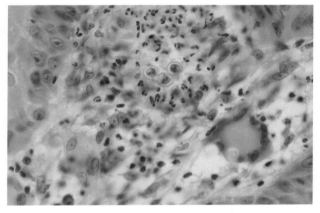

FIG. 16-7

Chromomycosis. The dermis shows an extensive infiltrate consisting of neutrophils and multinucleated giant cells. The causative organisms are found within giant cells. (× 40)

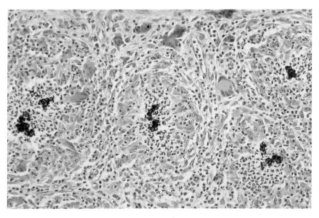

FIG. 16-8

Chromomycosis, higher magnification. The causative organisms appear as conspicuous, dark-brown, thick-walled, ovoid or spheric spores within giant cells or free in the tissue. They lie either singly or in chains or clusters. (× 160)

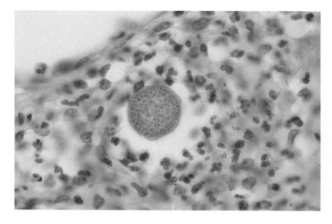

FIG. 16-9

Coccidioidomycosis. In the center of the picture a large spore containing endospores can be seen. Multiplication of the fungus takes place by forming endospores that are subsequently released into the tissue. The spore is surrounded by neutrophils and macrophages. (× 240)

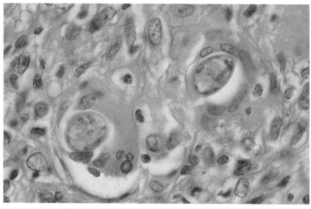

FIG. 16-10

Coccidioidomycosis. The spores of *Coccidioides immitis* vary greatly in size and are round and thick-walled. (× 240)

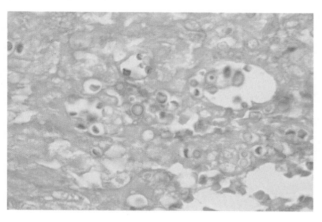

FIG. 16-11

Cryptococcosis, PAS stain, gelatinous lesion. Numerous organisms can be seen with only little tissue reaction. Each spore of *Cryptococcus neoformans* is surrounded by a wide gelatinous capsule. The capsule does not stain with hematoxylin or PAS. (× 240)

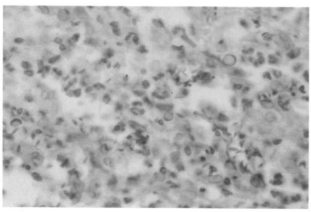

FIG. 16-12

Sporotrichosis, PAS stain. The spores of *Sporothrix schenckii* appear as round to oval bodies that stain more strongly at the periphery than in the center. (× 240)

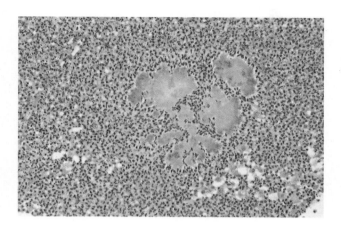

FIG. 16-13

Sulfur granule. A sulfur granule is lobulated, stains basophilic, and is surrounded by closely attached neutrophils. They can be found in actinomycosis, mycetoma, and botryomycosis. ($\times$ 64)

CHAPTER 17

Diseases Caused by Protozoa

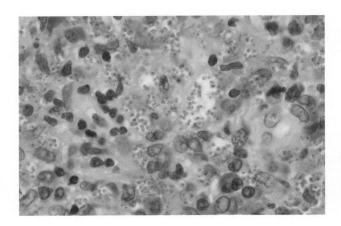

FIG. 17-1

Oriental leishmaniasis, H&E stain. Numerous leishmania organisms can be found within macrophages. The organisms can only be found during the first few months of the lesion. (× 240)

CHAPTER 18

Diseases Caused by Viruses

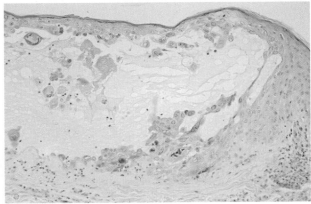

FIG. 18-1

Viral vesicles. An intraepidermal vesicle has formed owing to degeneration of epidermal cells, resulting in acantholysis. There is marked ballooning degeneration at the roof and the floor of the vesicle. Reticular degeneration is seen on the right side of the picture. ($\times$ 40)

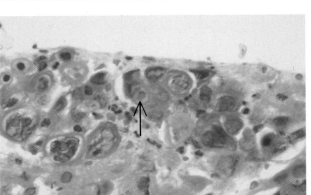

FIG. 18-2

Viral vesicle. Balloon cells at the floor of a vesicle are seen. Because the balloon cells lose their intercellular bridges, acantholysis occurs. An eosinophilic inclusion body (arrow) surrounded by a halo lies in the nucleus of a balloon cell. ($\times$ 160)

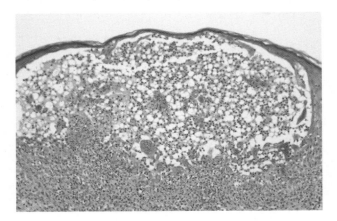

FIG. 18-3

Viral vesicles containing several multinucleated giant cells. This is an older viral vesicle that has been infiltrated by neutrophils. ($\times$ 40)

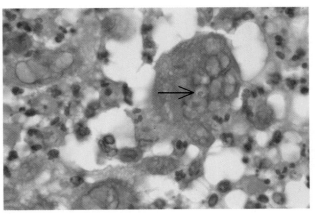

FIG. 18-4

Viral vesicle, higher magnification. Two multinucleated giant cells can be seen. An eosinophilic inclusion body surrounded by a halo lies in a nucleus of the giant cell in the center of the micrograph (arrow). ($\times$ 240)

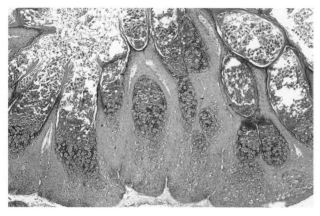

FIG. 18-5

Molluscum contagiosum. The epidermis consists of multiple lobules. Many epidermal cells contain large intracytoplasmic inclusion bodies. (× 16)

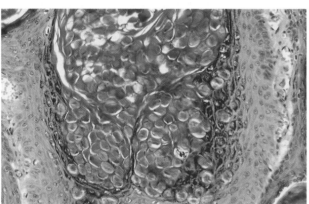

FIG. 18-6

Molluscum contagiosum, higher magnification. Numerous intracytoplasmic inclusion bodies, so-called molluscum bodies, can be seen. (× 64)

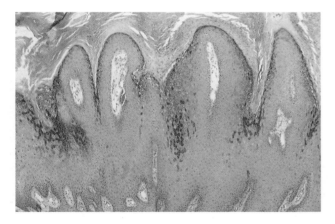

FIG. 18-7

Verruca vulgaris. The epidermis shows acanthosis, papillomatosis, hyperkeratosis. Within the granular layer perinuclear vacuolization can be seen. (× 16)

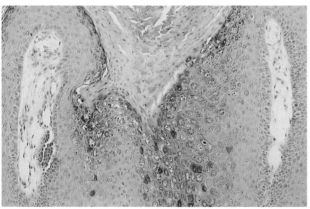

FIG. 18-8

Verruca vulgaris. The stratum corneum is parakeratotic. The granular cells show perinuclear edema and clumping of keratohyalin granules. (× 40)

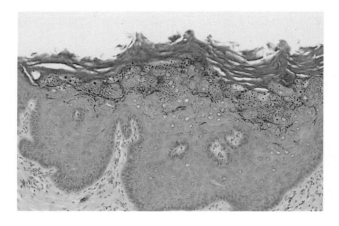

FIG. 18-9

Verruca plana. The epidermis shows acanthosis and hyperkeratosis. Perinuclear vacuolization is visible in the granular layer. (× 40)

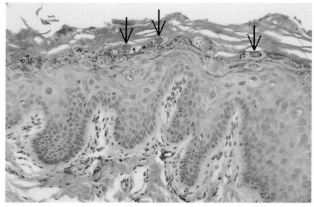

FIG. 18-10

Verruca plana. Incubation with a polyclonal antibody against papillomavirus antigen. A positive reaction can be seen in several nuclei (arrows) of the granular layer. (× 64)

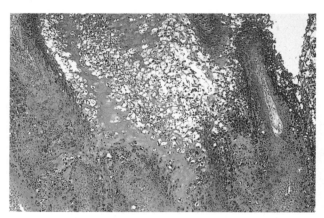

FIG. 18-11

Deep palmoplantar wart (myrmecia). The nuclei of the cells in the parakeratotic stratum corneum and in the granular cell layer are round, deeply basophilic, and surrounded by a clear zone. The deeply basophilic nuclei contain virus particles. (× 16)

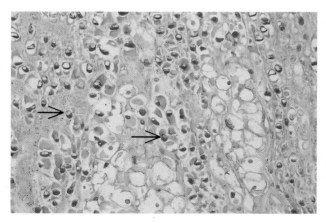

FIG. 18-12

Deep palmoplantar wart (myrmecia), incubation with papillomavirus antibody. The nuclei show a positive reaction (arrows). The cytoplasm of many cells contains large, irregularly shaped, homogeneous inclusions consisting of keratohyalin. (× 64)

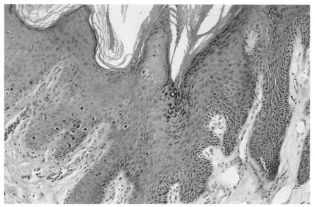

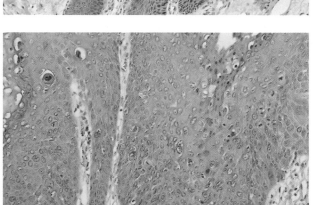

FIG. 18-13

Bowenoid papulosis. The epidermis shows acanthosis and hyperkeratosis. Several keratinocytes with hyperchromatic nuclei can be seen. (× 40)

FIG. 18-14

Bowenoid papulosis, higher magnification. Several dyskeratotic keratinocytes with atypical hyperchromatic nuclei can be seen. (× 64)

CHAPTER 19

Lipidoses

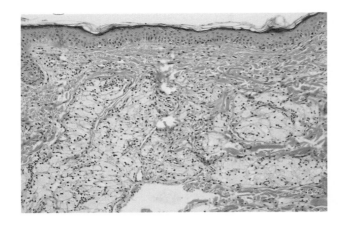

FIG. 19-1

Xanthelasma. In the upper dermis, islands of fat cells can be seen. (× 40)

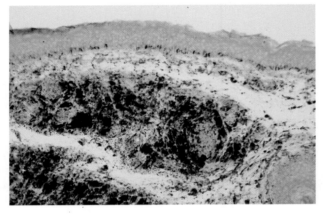

FIG. 19-2

Xanthelasma, Sudan black stain for fat. The foam cells are filled with lipid material. (× 40)

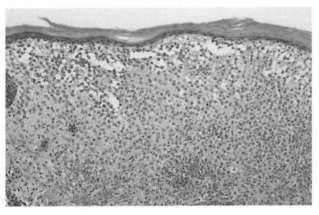

FIG. 19-3

Histiocytosis X, proliferative reaction. This reaction is typical for Letterer-Siwe disease and shows in the upper portion of the dermis an infiltrate composed almost exclusively of macrophages (Langerhans cells). They have invaded the epidermis and destroyed parts of it. (× 40)

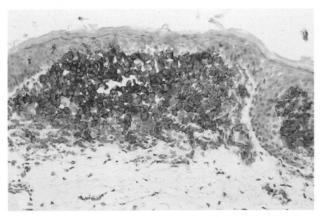

FIG. 19-4

Histiocytosis X, Letterer-Siwe disease. This cryostat section has been incubated with Leu 6, a monoclonal antibody directed against Langerhans cells. The infiltrate in the upper dermis consists almost exclusively of Langerhans cells. (× 64)

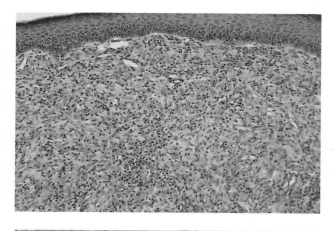

FIG. 19-5

Juvenile xanthogranuloma, early lesion. There are large accumulations of macrophages intermingled with a few lymphocytes in the upper dermis. The macrophages have a pale cytoplasm. (× 40)

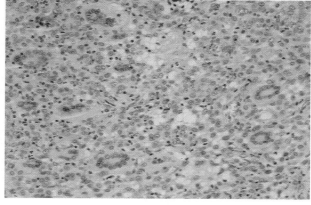

FIG. 19-6

Juvenile xanthogranuloma, mature lesion. A granulomatous infiltrate is present, consisting of foam cells, lymphocytes, and giant cells. Most of the giant cells show a perfect "wreath" of nuclei and peripheral to this "wreath," foamy cytoplasm. These so-called Touton giant cells are quite typical for juvenile xanthogranuloma. (× 64)

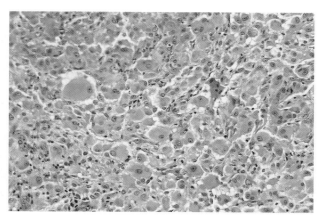

FIG. 19-7

Reticulohistiocytosis. Numerous large macrophages with abundant eosinophilic cytoplasm are present in the dermis. The cytoplasm has a ground-glass appearance. (× 64)

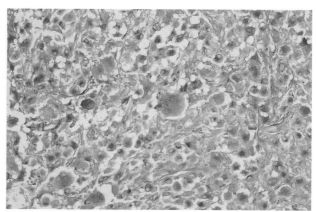

FIG. 19-8

Reticulohistiocytosis, PAS stain. The cytoplasm of the large macrophages is PAS positive and diastase resistant. (× 64)

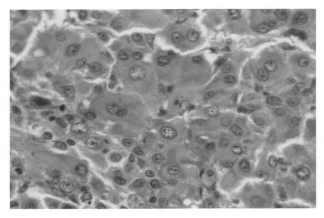

FIG. 19-9

Reticulohistiocytosis, higher magnification. Several of the large macrophages, with the ground-glass appearance of the cytoplasm, have more than one nucleus. (× 160)

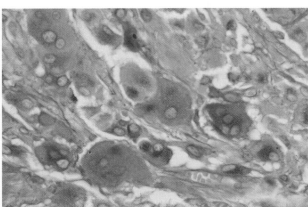

FIG. 19-10

Reticulohistiocytosis, PAS stain, higher magnification. The cytoplasm of the macrophages is strongly PAS positive and diastase resistant. (× 160)

CHAPTER 20

Metabolic
Diseases

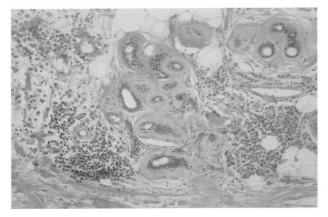

FIG. 20-1

Primary systemic amyloidosis. Amorphous, eosinophilic masses of amyloid are seen in the membrane propria surrounding the sweat glands. (× 40)

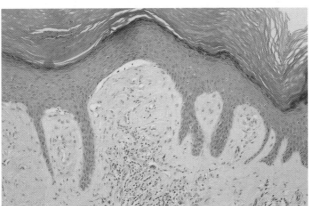

FIG. 20-2

Lichenoid amyloidosis. The epidermis shows acanthosis and hyperkeratosis. Amyloid is deposited in the papillae. It does not extend beyond the subpapillary plexus. (× 40)

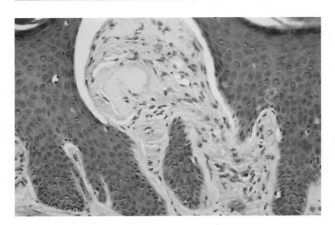

FIG. 20-3

Lichenoid amyloidosis, Congo red stain for the identification of amyloid. In lesions in which amyloid has only partially filled the papillae, the amyloid has a globular appearance. (× 64)

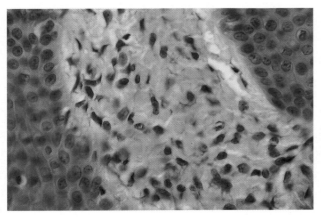

FIG. 20-4

Lichenoid amyloidosis, Congo red stain. The amyloid has a globular appearance, resembling colloid bodies. The amyloid-containing globular structures are degenerated epidermal cells. (× 160)

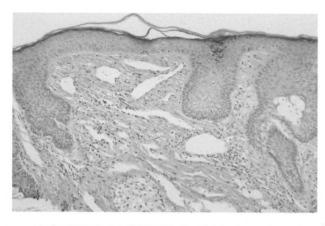

FIG. 20-5

Lichenoid amyloidosis, Congo red stain. The entire dermal papillae are filled with amyloid, which stains orange-red. ($\times$ 40)

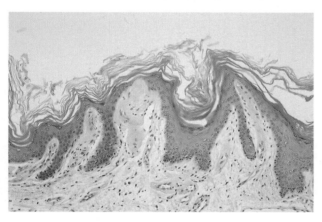

FIG. 20-6

Lichenoid amyloidosis, Congo red stain viewed in a polarizing light, similar section as Fig. 20-5. The amyloid shows greenish birefringence. ($\times$ 40)

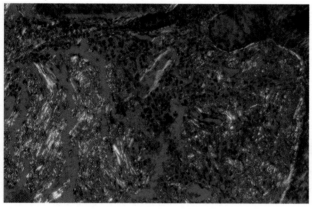

FIG. 20-7

Hyalinosis cutis et mucosae. Beneath a hyperkeratotic epidermis, a homogeneous, eosinophilic hyalin mantle surrounds the vessels throughout the dermis. ($\times$ 16)

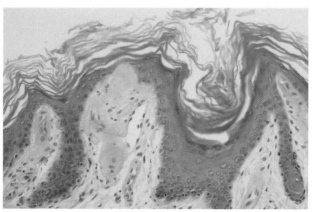

FIG. 20-8

Hyalinosis cutis et mucosae. Homogeneous eosinophilic hyalin material surrounds the blood vessels in the dermal papillae. ($\times$ 40)

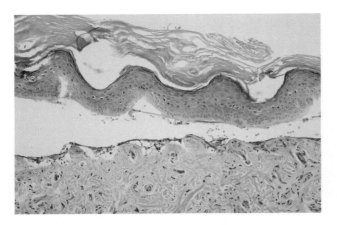

FIG. 20-9

Porphyria cutanea tarda. A subepidermal bulla is seen. The dermal papillae extend irregularly from the floor of the blister into the blister cavity. The blister has arisen above the basement membrane zone. (× 40)

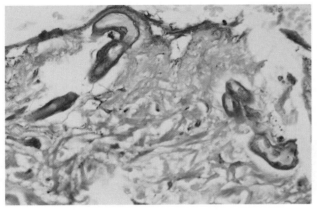

FIG. 20-10

Porphyria cutanea tarda, PAS stain. The capillaries in the dermis show a thick mantle of PAS-positive material around them. (× 160)

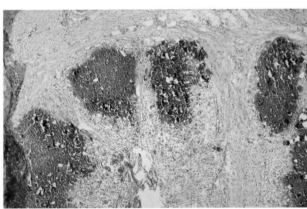

FIG. 20-11

Idiopathic calcinosis cutis. Calcium deposits stain bluish-red with H&E. They are surrounded by fibrosis. (× 16)

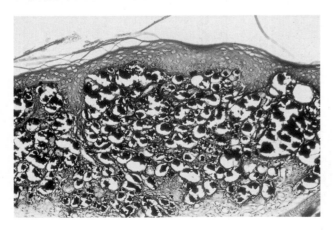

FIG. 20-12

Subepidermal calcified nodule, von Kossa stain for calcium. The calcium is present as closely aggregated globules, which are black. (× 40)

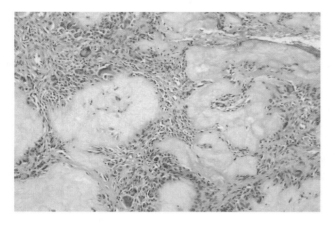

FIG. 20-13

Gout, formalin fixation. Amorphous material consisting of urates is surrounded by macrophages and foreign body giant cells. (× 40)

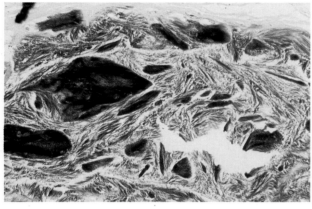

FIG. 20-14

Gout, von Kossa stain, fixation in alcohol. Urate crystals lie closely packed in the form of bundles. The crystals have a brownish color. As a secondary phenomenon, calcification has occurred. (× 40)

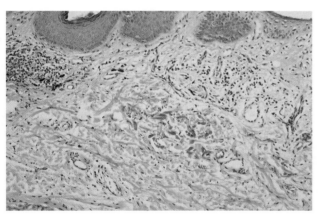

FIG. 20-15

Ochronosis. The ochronotic pigment stains yellow brown in H&E stains. The ochronotic pigment is located within collagen bundles. (× 40)

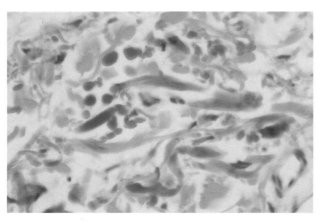

FIG. 20-16

Ochronosis, higher magnification. The yellow brown ochronotic pigment is present within collagen bundles, causing homogenization and swelling of the bundles. The collagen bundles appear rigid and tend to fracture. As the result of the breaking up, irregular, homogeneous, light brown clumps lie free in the tissue. (× 160)

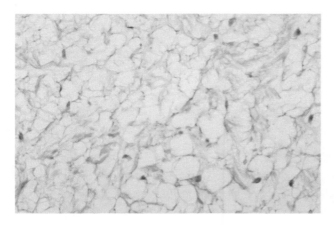

FIG. 20-17

Pretibial myxedema. Mucin is present in large amounts in the dermis. It appears stringy and to lie in empty spaces owing to shrinkage during the process of fixation and dehydration. A few stellate-shaped fibroblasts (mucoblasts) are seen between the mucin. (× 64)

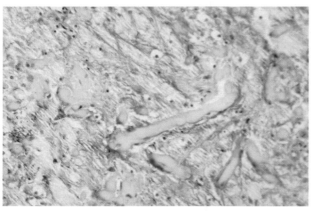

FIG. 20-18

Pretibial myxedema, methylene blue stain. This stains mucin metachromatically, which thus appears purple rather than blue. (× 40)

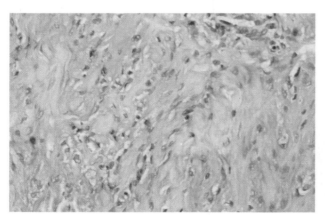

FIG. 20-19

Scleromyxedema (lichen myxedematosus), alcian blue stain. Mucin and mucoblasts stain blue. In addition to fairly large amounts of mucin (blue), there is extensive proliferation of fibroblasts (red). (× 64)

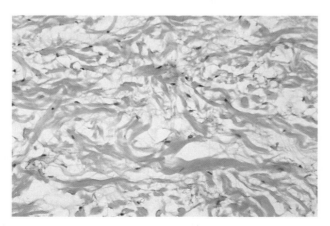

FIG. 20-20

Reticular erythematous mucinosis (REM syndrome). Mucinous deposits are visible as threats and streaks between collagen bundles in routinely stained sections. (× 40)

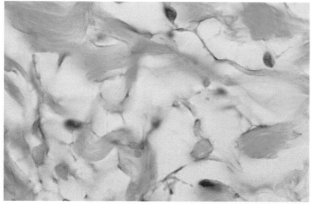

FIG. 20-21

Reticular erythematous mucinosis (REM syndrome), higher magnification. Mucinous material can be seen as threads between collagen bundles. ($\times$ 160)

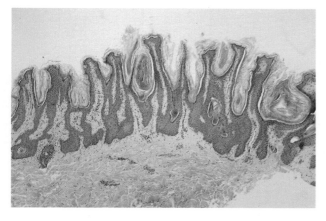

FIG. 20-22

Reticular erythematous mucinosis (REM syndrome), alcian stain. The mucinous material appears as blue threads. ($\times$ 240)

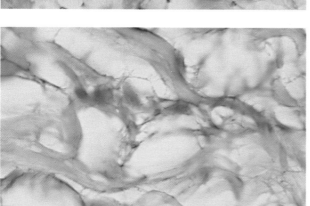
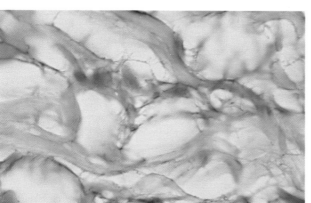

FIG. 20-23

Acanthosis nigricans. There is hyperkeratosis and papillomatosis, but only slight acanthosis and no hyperpigmentation. The dermal papillae project upward as fingerlike projections. The valleys between the papillae are filled with keratotic material. ($\times$ 16)

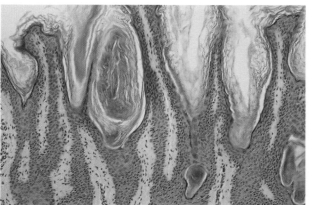

FIG. 20-24

Acanthosis nigricans. The stratum malpighii at the tips and on the sides of the protruding papillae appears thinned. There is no hyperpigmentation. The brownish color of the lesions thus is caused by hyperkeratosis rather than by melanin. ($\times$ 40)

CHAPTER 21

Connective
Tissue
Diseases

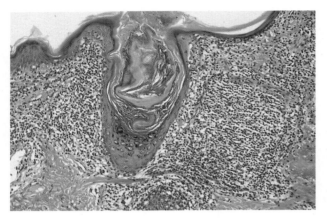

FIG. 21-1

Lupus erythematosus. The epidermis is atrophic, the hair follicle shows keratotic plugging. Subepidermally a dense lymphocytic infiltrate can be seen. (× 40)

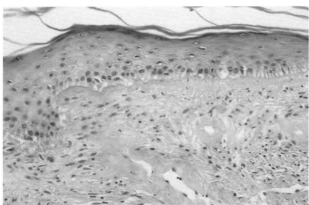

FIG. 21-2

Lupus erythematosus. The basal cells show hydropic degeneration. The epidermis appears rather flat. (× 64)

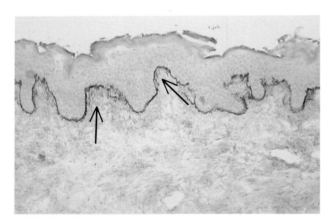

FIG. 21-3

Lupus erythematosus, direct immunoperoxidase of uninvolved skin. At the dermal-epidermal junction a linear band of immunoglobulins is seen. In contrast to the band in bullous pemphigoid, the band in lupus erythematosus shows irregular extensions into the uppermost dermis (arrows). (× 40)

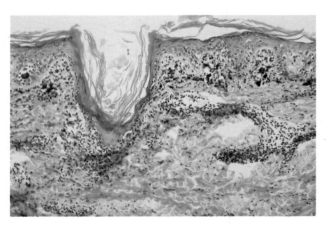

FIG. 21-4

Lupus erythematosus. The hair follicle is dilated and shows keratotic plugging. The epidermis is thinned. Because of liquefaction degeneration of the basal cell layer, there is considerable pigmentary incontinence in the upper dermis. (× 40)

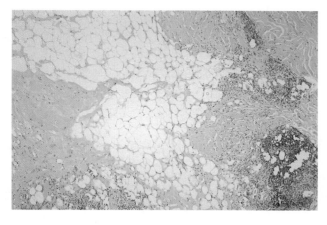

FIG. 21-5

Lupus erythematosus profundus. The subcutaneous fat has been partially replaced by homogeneous, glassy, eosinophilic collagen. On the right side of the photomicrograph infiltrates of lymphoid cells are seen. (× 16)

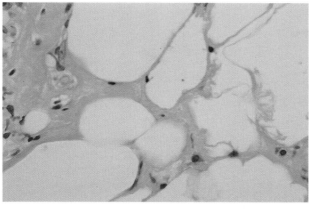

FIG. 21-6

Lupus erythematosus profundus. Hyalinized collagen is seen to separate individual fat cells from one another. (× 160)

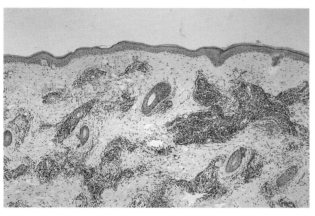

FIG. 21-7

Jessner's lymphocytic infiltration. The epidermis is slightly flattened. In the dermis, fairly well circumscribed patches of a cellular infiltrate are seen consisting almost entirely of lymphocytes. (× 16)

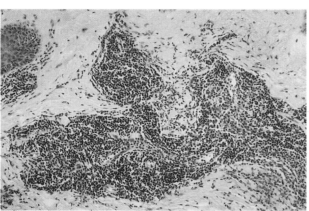

FIG. 21-8

Jessner's lymphocytic infiltration, higher magnification. The infiltrate is seen around blood vessels. It mainly consists of lymphocytes with a few macrophages mixed in. (× 40)

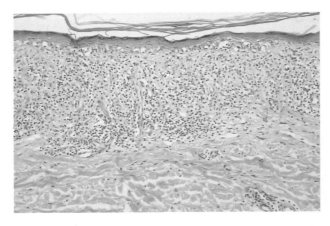

FIG. 21-9

Poikiloderma atrophicans vasculare in lupus erythematosus. The epidermis shows thinning of the stratum malpighii with marked hydropic degeneration of the basal cells. Subepidermally a dense bandlike infiltrate of mononuclear cells is seen. (× 40)

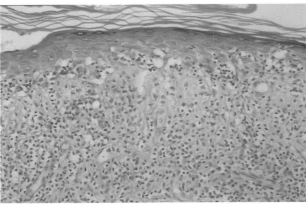

FIG. 21-10

Poikiloderma atrophicans vasculare in lupus erythematosus, higher magnification. The epidermis is flattened and shows hydropic degeneration of the basal cells. The upper dermis shows a bandlike infiltrate consisting of lymphocytes. The lymphocytes have invaded the lower part of the epidermis. (× 64)

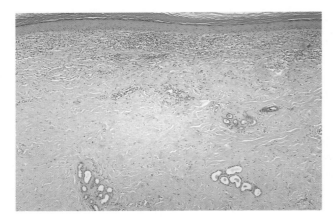

FIG. 21-11

Scleroderma. The epidermis is flat, the upper dermis shows an inflammatory infiltrate. The collagen appears thickened and closely packed. The eccrine glands are surrounded by newly formed collagen instead of by fat cells. Owing to thickening of the dermis, they seem to be located within the dermis rather than at the junction between dermis and subcutaneous fat. (× 16)

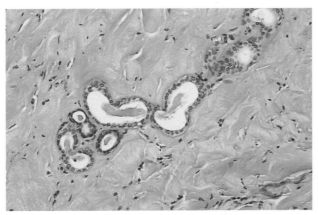

FIG. 21-12

Scleroderma. The eccrine glands are atrophic and appear tightly bound-down by newly formed collagen. (× 64)

C H A P T E R 22

Tumors and Cysts of the Epidermis

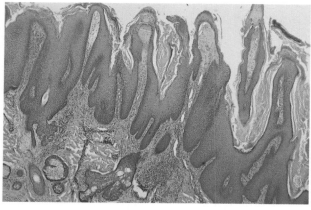

FIG. 22-1

Epidermal nevus. There is hyperkeratosis, papillomatosis, and acanthosis with elongation of the rete ridges. This is the histologic picture of a benign papilloma. (× 16)

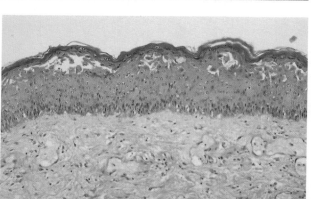

FIG. 22-2

Solitary epidermolytic acanthoma. In the upper stratum malpighii acantholysis is seen. (× 40)

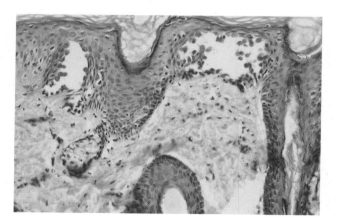

FIG. 22-3

Incidental focal acantholytic dyskeratosis. There are focal suprabasal clefts. (× 64)

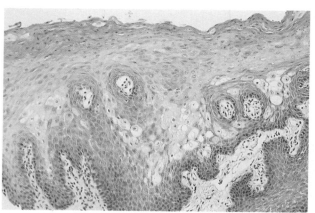

FIG. 22-4

Oral white sponge nevus. The oral mucosa shows hyperplasia with much more pronounced hydropic swelling of the epithelial cells than is seen in normal oral mucosa. The hydropic swelling is focal. (× 40)

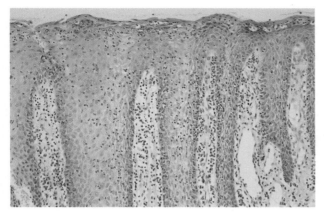

FIG. 22-5

Lingua geographica. The mucosa shows acanthosis with elongation of the rete ridges and permeation by neutrophils. There is no granular layer, which is normally present on the dorsum of the tongue. (× 40)

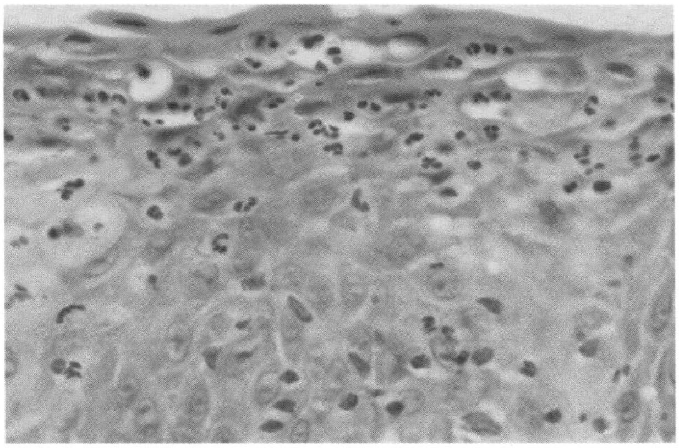

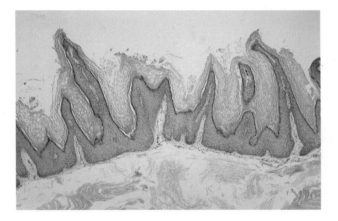

FIG. 22-6

Lingua geographica, higher magnification. In the upper portion of the mucosa, neutrophils are present in the interstices of a spongelike network of degenerated keratinocytes. The histologic picture thus shows similar to psoriasis Kogoj's spongiform pustules. (× 160)

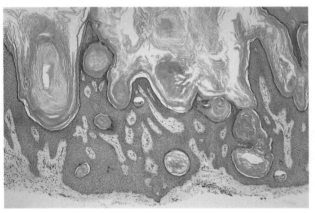

FIG. 22-7

Seborrheic keratosis, hyperkeratotic type. The epidermis shows acanthosis and hyperkeratosis. The upward extensions of epidermis-lined papillae have been compared to church spires. (× 16)

FIG. 22-8

Seborrheic keratosis, acanthotic type. The epidermis shows acanthosis with papillomatosis and hyperkeratosis. Horny invaginations are seen, which on cross section appear as pseudo-horn cysts. In addition, true horn cysts are seen, which show sudden and complete keratinization. (× 16)

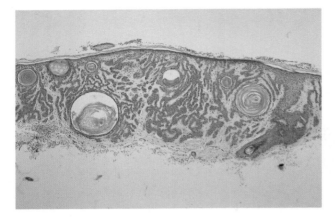

FIG. 22-9

Seborrheic keratosis, adenoid type. Numerous thin tracts of epidermal cells extend from the epidermis and show branching and interweaving in the dermis. Several horn cysts are present. (× 16)

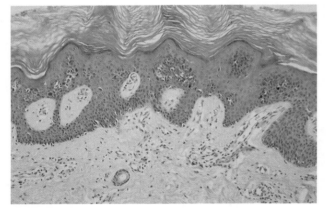

FIG. 22-10

Seborrheic keratosis, adenoid type, higher magnification. Thin tracts composed of a double row of basaloid cells extend from the epidermis into the dermis. (× 40)

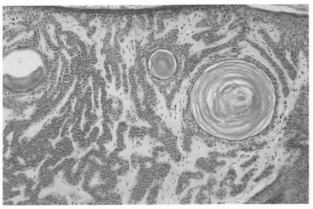

FIG. 22-11

Seborrheic keratosis, pigmented type (melanoacanthoma). The epidermis shows hyperpigmentation, slightly acanthosis, and groups of pigmented melanocytes. (× 40)

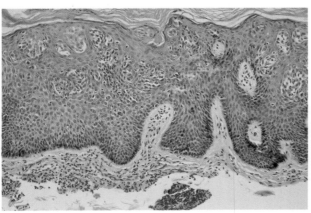

FIG. 22-12

Seborrheic keratosis, pigmented type (melanoacanthoma). The basal cell layer is hyperpigmented, and within the epidermis groups of pigmented melanocytes are seen. (× 40)

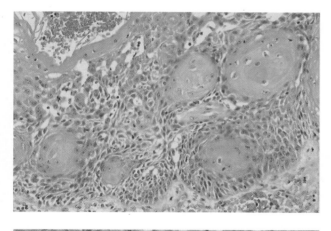

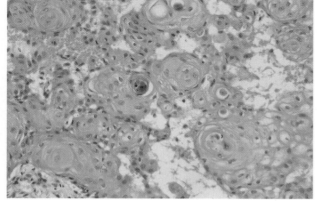

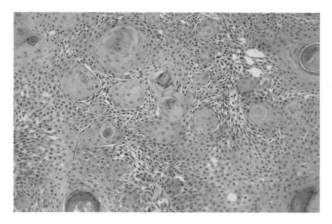

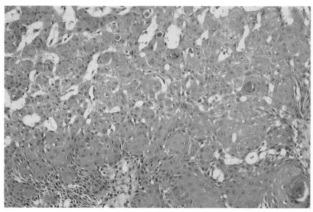

FIG. 22·13 through FIG. 22·16

Seborrheic keratosis, irritated type. Numerous whorls or eddies are present that are composed of eosinophilic flattened squamous cells arranged in an onion peel fashion, resembling poorly differentiated horn pearls. In contrast to the horn pearls in squamous cell carcinoma, these "squamous eddies" are small in size, circumscribed in configuration, and numerous. (Fig. 22-13, Fig. 22-14 × 64; Fig 22-15, Fig. 22-16 × 40)

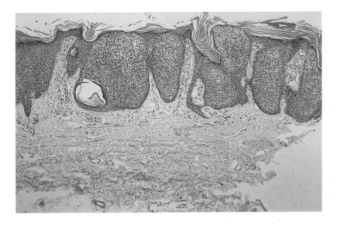

FIG. 22-17

Seborrheic keratosis, clonal or nesting type. Well-defined nests of keratinocytes are located within the epidermis. (× 16)

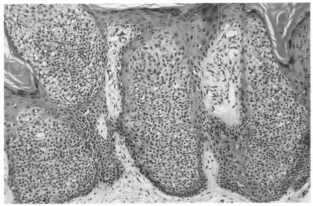

FIG. 22-18

Seborrheic keratosis, clonal type, higher magnification of Fig. 22-17. Large, well-defined nests of keratinocytes are present in the epidermis. (× 40)

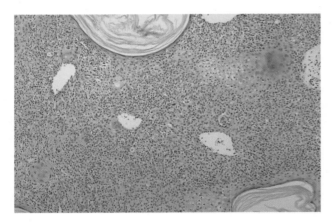

FIG. 22-19

Seborrheic keratosis with features of Bowen's disease. Several large atypical keratinocytes are present, as well as horn cysts. (× 16)

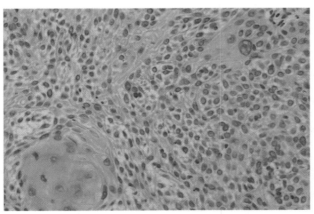

FIG. 22-20

Seborrheic keratosis with features of Bowen's disease, higher magnification of Fig. 22-19. A horn pearl is present on the left side of the photomicrograph and atypical keratinocytes, on the right side. (× 64)

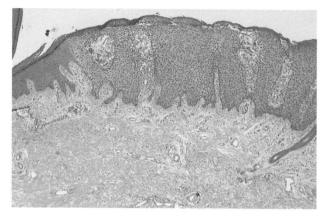

FIG. 22-21

Clear cell acanthoma. Within a sharply demarcated area of the epidermis, all keratinocytes except for basal keratinocytes appear strikingly clear. (× 16)

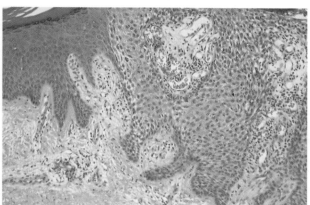

FIG. 22-22

Clear cell acanthoma, higher magnification of Fig. 22-21. There is a sharp border between the keratinocytes of normal epidermis and those of the clear cell acanthoma. (× 40)

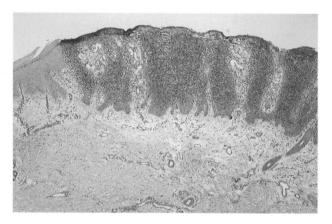

FIG. 22-23

Clear cell acanthoma, PAS stain. The clarity of the cytoplasm of the keratinocytes within the clear cell acanthoma is due to large accumulations of glycogen, which stains red with PAS. (× 16)

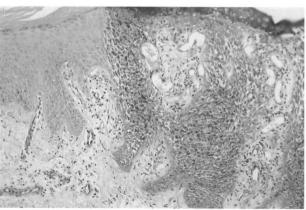

FIG. 22-24

Clear cell acanthoma, PAS stain, higher magnification. Whereas the keratinocytes in the normal epidermis do not stain with PAS, the cytoplasm of the cells in clear cell acanthoma stains positively with PAS, owing to an accumulation of glycogen. (× 40)

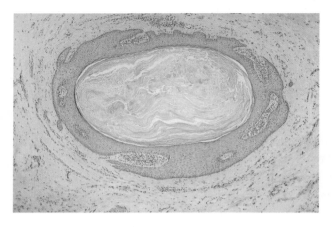

FIG. 22-25

Small epidermal cyst (milium). The wall is composed of true epidermis, as seen on the skin surface and in the infundibulum of hair follicles. The cyst is filled with horny material arranged in laminated layers. (× 16)

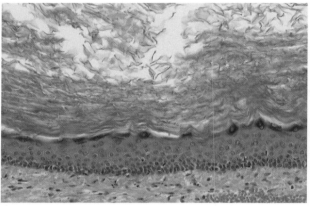

FIG. 22-26

Epidermal cyst. The wall of the cyst is composed of true epidermis: squamous, granular, and horn cells. The cyst is filled with horny material that looks like "shredded wheat." (× 64)

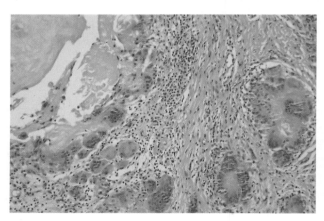

FIG. 22-27

Ruptured epidermal cyst. In the left upper corner some horny material is present. The cyst wall has disintegrated. A foreign body reaction of multinucleated giant cells is present. (× 40)

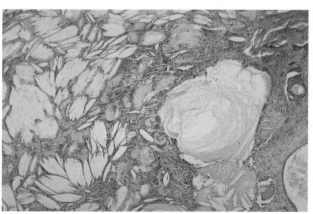

FIG. 22-28

Ruptured epidermal cyst with cholesterol crystals. The cholesterol crystals are intermingled with foreign body giant cells. (× 16)

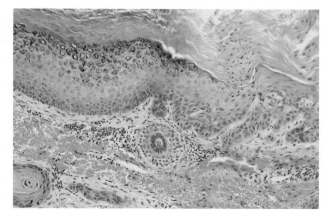

FIG. 22-29

Epidermal cyst with malignant degeneration. On the left side normal epidermis is seen. On the right side of the photomicrograph parakeratosis with absence of a granular layer is seen, and there is a proliferation of strands of keratinocytes into the dermis. (× 40)

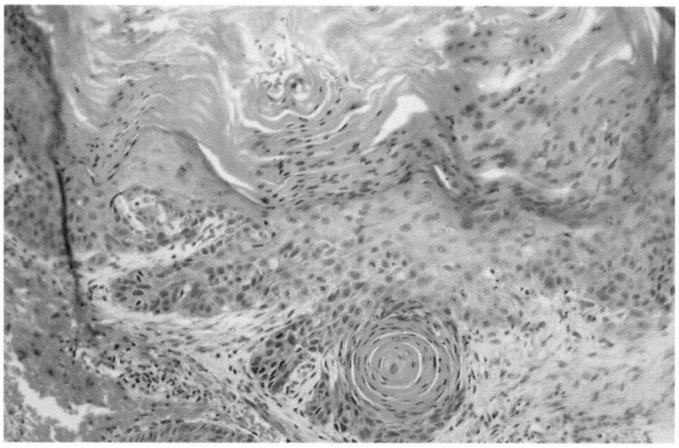

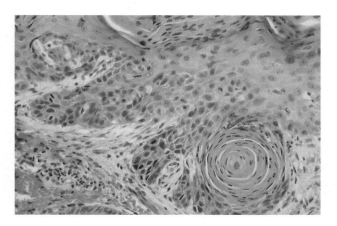

FIG. 22-30

Epidermal cyst with squamous cell carcinoma in its wall. The cyst wall shows acanthosis and a horn pearl. The orderly arrangement of the keratinocytes is gone. (× 40)

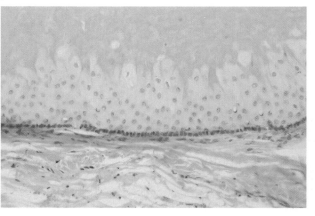

FIG. 22-31

Epidermal cyst with squamous cell carcinoma in its wall. The nuclei of most keratinocytes are large. A horn pearl can be seen consisting of concentric layers of parakeratotic cells. (× 64)

FIG. 22-32

Trichilemmal cyst. The peripheral cell layer of the cyst wall shows distinct palisading. The cells close to the cystic cavity are swollen. The lumen of the cyst is filled with homogeneous material. (× 64)

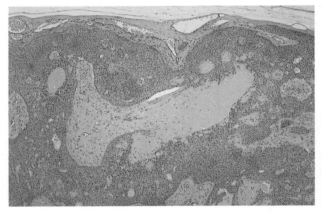

FIG. 22-33

Proliferating trichilemmal cyst. The lesion is well demarcated from the surrounding tissue and consists of lobules composed of squamous epithelium. The epithelium in the center of the lobules abruptly changes into amorphous keratin. ($\times$ 16)

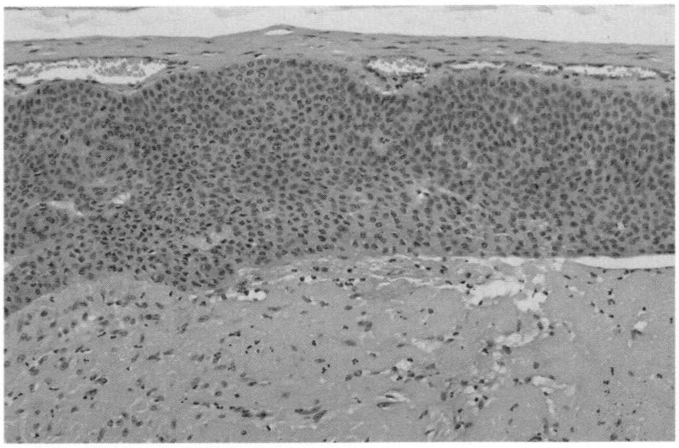

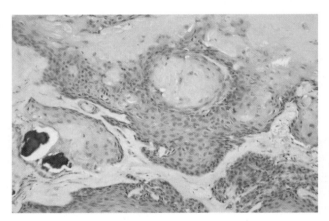

FIG. 22-34

Proliferating trichilemmal cyst, higher magnification of the cyst wall. The peripheral cell layer shows palisading. The cyst is surrounded by a vitreous layer. The lumen is filled with amorphous keratin. ($\times$ 40)

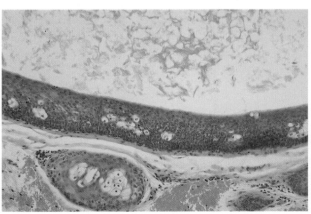

FIG. 22-35

Proliferating trichilemmal cyst with some calcification. The lesion is composed of irregularly shaped lobules of squamous epithelium. On the left side a small focus of calcification is present. ($\times$ 40)

FIG. 22-36

Steatocystoma multiplex. The cyst wall consists of several layers of epithelial cells. Sebaceous gland cells are present within the cyst wall. A flattened sebaceous gland lobule is present close to the cyst wall. ($\times$ 40)

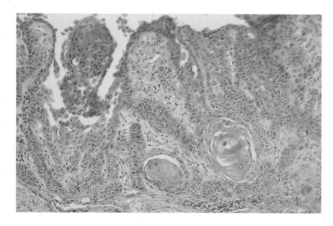

FIG. 22-37

Warty dyskeratoma. The lesion shows a cup-shaped invagination in which numerous acantholytic cells are present. The lower portion of the invagination is occupied by numerous villi. The latter are elongated dermal papillae that project upward. (× 40)

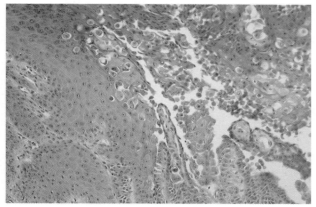

FIG. 22-38

Warty dyskeratoma, higher magnification. The cup-shaped invagination is filled with dyskeratotic, acantholytic cells. Several corps ronds are visible in the thickened granular layer lining the wall of the cup-shaped invagination. The villi present at the base of the invagination are lined by a single layer of basal cells. (× 64)

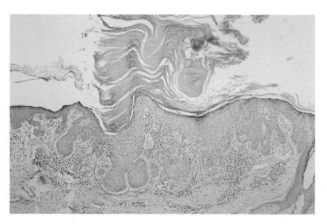

FIG. 22-39

Cornu cutaneum with an underlying solar keratosis. The cutaneous horn consists of layers of parakeratotic cells. The underlying epidermis shows irregular buds extending into the dermis. (× 16)

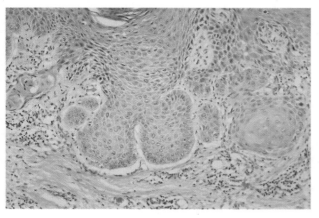

FIG. 22-40

Solar keratosis, higher magnification of Fig. 22-39. The irregular buds that extend from the epidermis into the dermis show pleomorphic, atypical nuclei. (× 40)

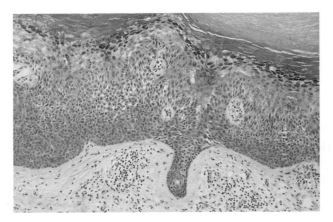

FIG. 22-41

Solar keratosis with epidermolytic hyperkeratosis. The stratum granulosum is thickened and shows clear spaces around the nuclei. The keratinocytes show a disorderly arrangement within the epidermis. (× 40)

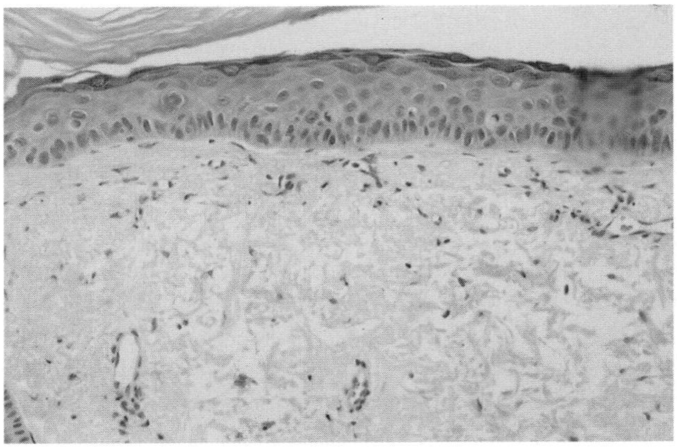

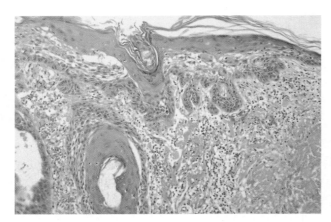

FIG. 22-42

Solar keratosis, atrophic type. The epidermis is atrophic and devoid of rete ridges. Atypical cells are found in the basal cell layer and directly above it. The atypical cells have large hyperchromatic nuclei that lie close together. (× 40)

FIG. 22-43

Solar keratosis, acantholytic type. Above the atypical cells composing the basal cell layer, clefts or lacunae are seen. These clefts form because of anaplastic changes in the lowermost epidermis, resulting in dyskeratosis and loss of intercellular bridges. (× 40)

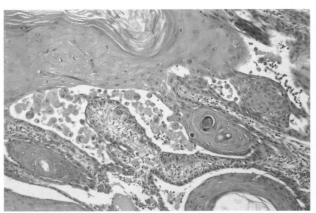

FIG. 22-44

Solar keratosis, acantholytic type, higher magnification. Clefts or lacunae have formed above the basal layer. Within the lacunae atypical dyskeratotic cells are seen. (× 64)

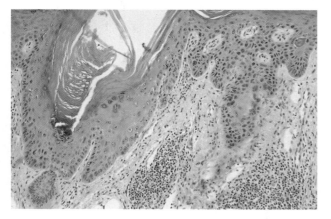

FIG. 22-45

Solar keratosis, bowenoid type, with early invasion. The epidermis shows irregular buds of atypical cells extending from the epidermis into the dermis. Some of the keratinocytes show hyperchromatic atypical nuclei. (× 40)

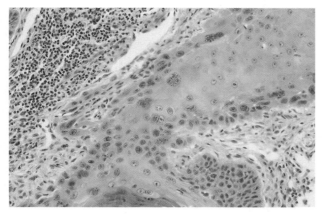

FIG. 22-46

Solar keratosis, bowenoid type, with early invasion, higher magnification. Within the epidermis considerable disorder in the arrangement of nuclei can be seen, as well as clumping of nuclei. (× 64)

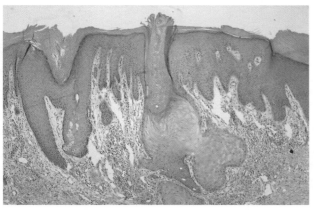

FIG. 22-47

Solar keratosis with early invasion. In the center of the hyperkeratotic lesion an invasion into the dermis has taken place. (× 16)

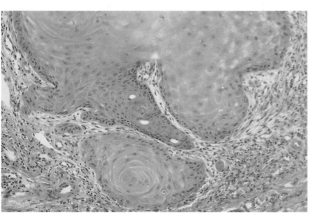

FIG. 22-48

Solar keratosis with early invasion, higher magnification of Fig. 22-47. At the bottom of the photomicrograph an island composed of atypical keratinocytes is located entirely in the dermis. (× 40)

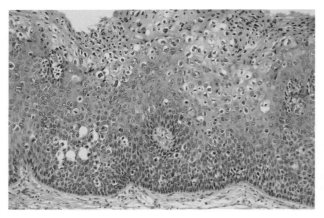

FIG. 22-49

Bowen's disease. The epidermis shows acanthosis. Throughout the epidermis the cells lie in complete disorder; many of them look atypical, showing hyperchromatic, large nuclei. (× 40)

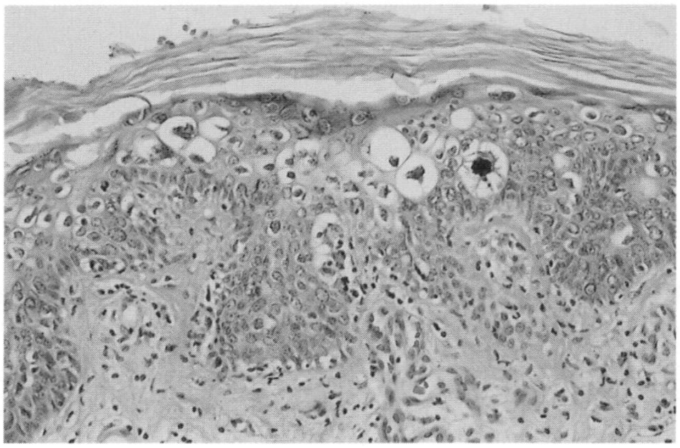

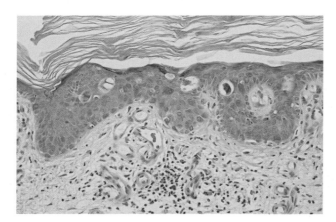

FIG. 22-50

Bowen's disease. The rete ridges are thickened and elongated. Within the epidermis atypical keratinocytes with hyperchromatic nuclei and a vacuolated cytoplasm can be seen. (× 64)

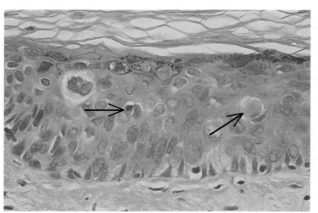

FIG. 22-51

Bowen's disease. Several of the atypical cells show vacuolization of the cytoplasm. (× 64)

FIG. 22-52

Bowen's disease. Within the thickened epidermis individual cell keratinization can be seen. These dyskeratotic cells have a strongly eosinophilic cytoplasm (arrows). On the left side of the photomicrograph a multinucleated atypical keratinocyte can be seen. (× 160)

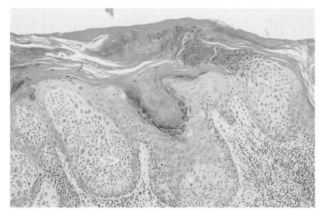

FIG. 22-53

Bowen's disease, clonal type. Nests of atypical keratinocytes are scattered through the epidermis. (× 40)

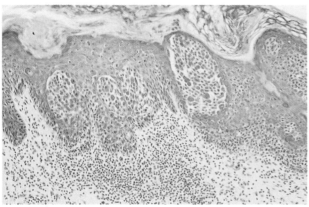

FIG. 22-54

Bowen's disease, clonal type. The section has been incubated with a monoclonal antibody against keratin. A positive reaction is present within the cytoplasm. (× 40)

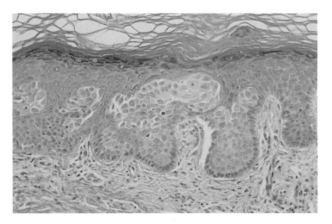

FIG. 22-55

Bowen's disease, clonal type. Atypical keratinocytes are arranged within well-defined nests within the epidermis. (× 64)

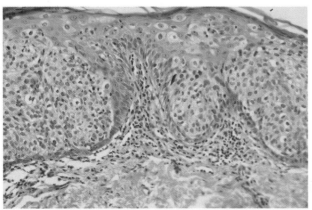

FIG. 22-56

Bowen's disease, clonal type. Nests of atypical keratinocytes are present within the epidermis. (× 64)

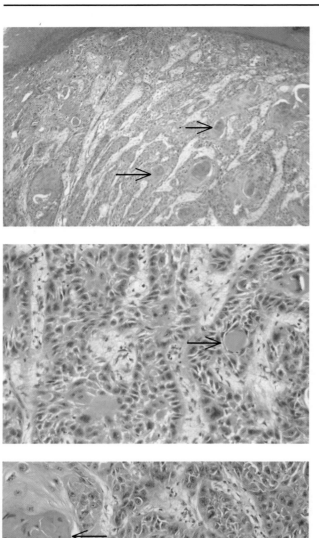

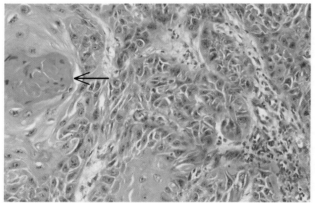

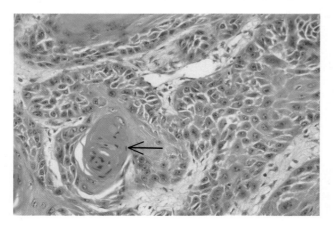

FIG. 22-57 through FIG. 22-60

Squamous cell carcinoma, well differentiated.
Within the dermis well-defined strands of atypical
keratinocytes can be seen. Within these strands horn
pearls (arrows) are seen composed of concentric layers of
squamous cells showing gradually increasing keratinization
toward the center. The invading tumor strands are composed in varying proportions of normal squamous cells and
of atypical (anaplastic) squamous cells. Atypicality ex-
presses itself as variation in the size and shape of the cells,
in hyperplasia and hyperchromasia of the nuclei and/or
in absence of intercellular bridges. (Fig. 22-57 × 16, Fig.
22-58 through Fig. 22-60 × 64).

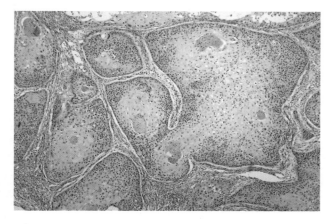

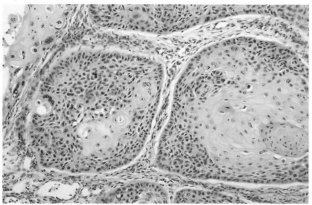

FIG. 22-61 and FIG. 22-62

Squamous cell carcinoma, well differentiated.
Within the dermis well-circumscribed islands of atypical keratinocytes are present. Within these islands several horn pearls are visible. (Fig. 22-61 × 16, Fig. 22-62 × 40)

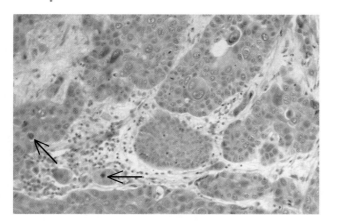

FIG. 22-63

Squamous cell carcinoma, well differentiated.
Within the dermis tumor islands of varying size are present. Within these islands dyskeratotic cells with hyperchromatic nuclei (arrows) are present. (× 40)

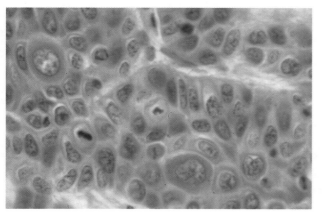

FIG. 22-64

Squamous cell carcinoma, well differentiated.
The atypical cells vary in size and shape and show a varying number of mitoses. (× 160)

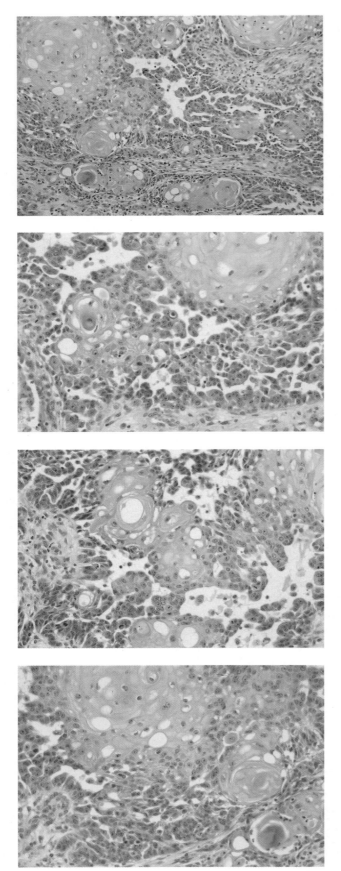

FIG. 22-65 through FIG. 22-68

Squamous cell carcinoma with acantholysis.
There is dyskeratosis with individual cell keratinization, resulting in acantholysis within a lobule. Formation of lumina results, which contain acantholytic cells. (Fig. 22-65 × 40; Fig. 22-66 through Fig. 22-68 × 64)

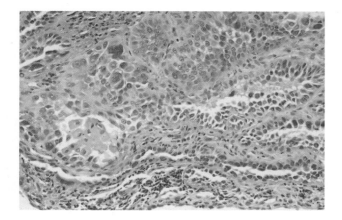

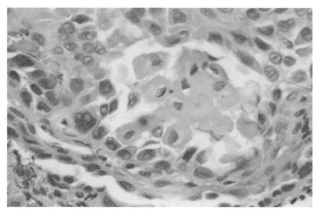

FIG. 22-69 and FIG. 22-70

Squamous cell carcinoma with dyskeratosis and acantholysis. Within the tumor islands a varying number of dyskeratotic cells with a strongly eosinophilic cytoplasm are seen (Fig. 22-70). (Fig. 22-69 × 64, Fig. 22-70 × 160)

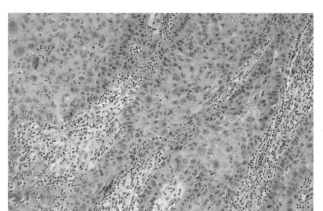

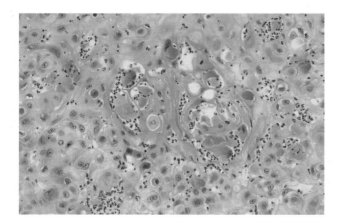

FIG. 22-71 and FIG. 22-72

Squamous cell carcinoma with marked dyskeratosis consisting of individual cell keratinization (Fig. 22-71) and groups of dyskeratotic cells. (Fig. 22-71 × 40, Fig. 22-72 × 64)

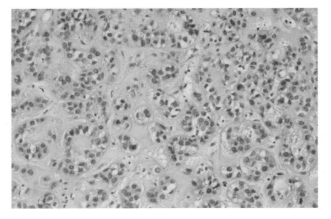

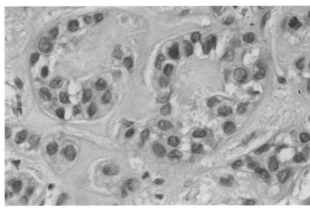

FIG. 22-73 and FIG. 22-74

Squamous cell carcinoma, undifferentiated.
Tubular strands are seen within the corium. The cells do not show any keratinization. The strands consist of two layers of keratinocytes. (Fig. 22-73 × 40, Fig. 22-74 × 64)

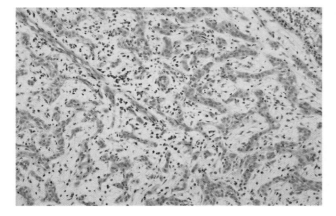

FIG. 22-75

Squamous cell carcinoma, undifferentiated.
Within the dermis strands of atypical basophilic cells are seen. There is no evidence of keratinization. (× 40)

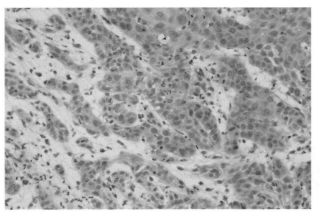

FIG. 22-76

Squamous cell carcinoma, undifferentiated, higher magnification of Fig. 22-75. Strands of atypical cells are seen to have infiltrated the dermis. (× 64)

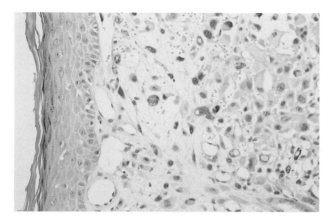

FIG. 22-77

Squamous cell carcinoma. Within the dermis atypical large keratinocytes are seen. The cells have large hyperchromatic nuclei. There are no intercellular bridges. The tumor resembles atypical fibroxanthoma on account of the giant cells. ($\times$ 64)

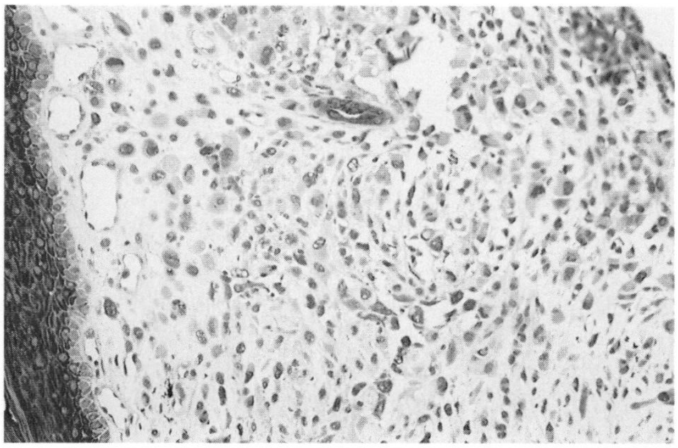

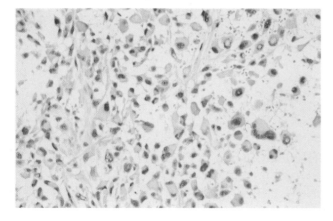

FIG. 22-78

Squamous cell carcinoma, incubation with a monoclonal antibody against keratin. Many of the atypical cells show a positive reaction product (red color). APAAP technique. ($\times$ 40)

FIG. 22-79

Squamous cell carcinoma, undifferentiated. The atypical cells have large, hyperchromatic nuclei. The tumor cells have lost the coherence to one another. ($\times$ 64)

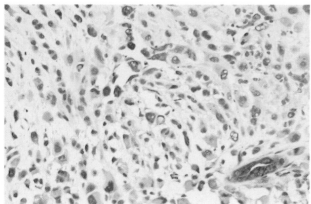

FIG. 22-80

Squamous cell carcinoma, undifferentiated, incubated with a monoclonal antibody against keratin. Most tumor cells show a positive reaction. Many of the atypical nuclei have vesicular nuclei. APAAP technique. ($\times$ 64)

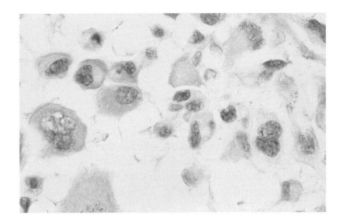

FIG. 22-81

Squamous cell carcinoma, incubated with a monoclonal antibody against keratin. Most of the tumor cells show a positive reaction (yellow-brown color). ABC technique. (× 240)

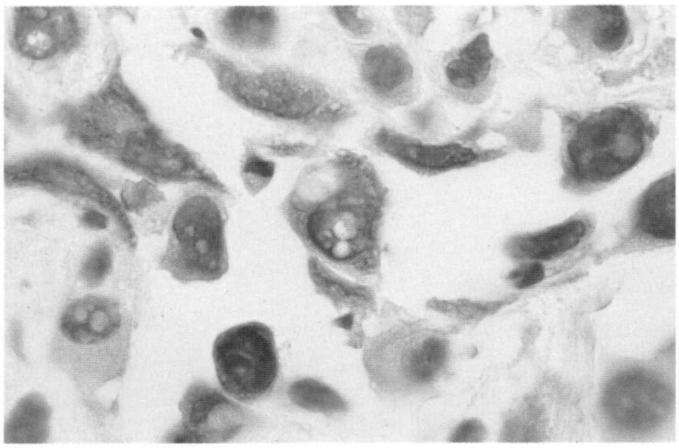

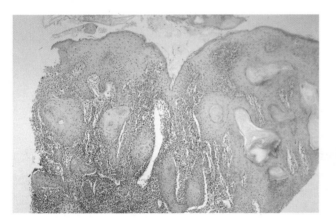

FIG. 22-82

Squamous cell carcinoma, incubation with a monoclonal antibody against keratin. The cytoplasm shows a positive reaction (red color). APAAP technique. The atypical cells have large hyperchromatic nuclei with vesicular nucleoli. (× 240)

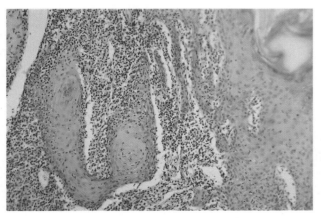

FIG. 22-83

Pseudocarcinomatous hyperplasia. The epidermis shows hyperplasia. Epidermal cell masses have invaded the dermis. The epidermal strands show horn pearl formation. (× 16)

FIG. 22-84

Pseudocarcinomatous hyperplasia, higher magnification. Within the dermis epidermal strands with horn pearls are seen. The cells are well differentiated. (× 40)

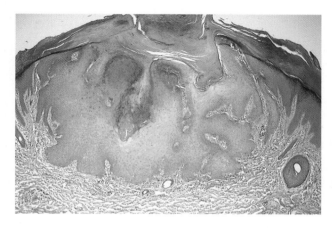

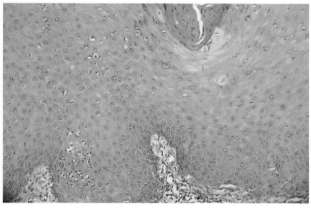

FIG. 22-85

Keratoacanthoma. A horn-filled crater is seen. The epidermis extends like a lip or buttress over the sides of the crater. At the base of the crater irregular epidermal proliferations extend both upward into the crater and downward into the dermis. The lesion is sharply demarcated. (× 10)

FIG. 22-86

Keratoacanthoma, higher magnification. The keratinocytes appear eosinophilic and glassy as a result of keratinization. (× 40)

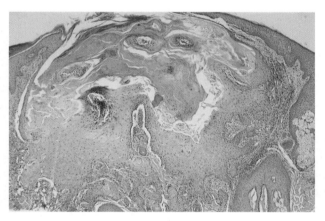

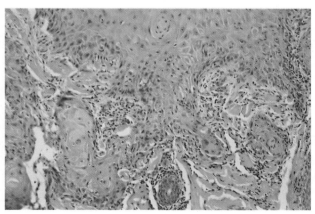

FIG. 22-87

Keratoacanthoma. The lesion shows a large crater that is filled with keratin. The epidermis extends like a lip over the sides of the crater. This lesion is poorly demarcated from the surrounding dermis. (× 10)

FIG. 22-88

Keratoacanthoma. The base of the tumor shows a poor demarcation from the surrounding dermis. The tumor cells show good keratinization, which gives them an eosinophilic, glassy appearance. (× 40)

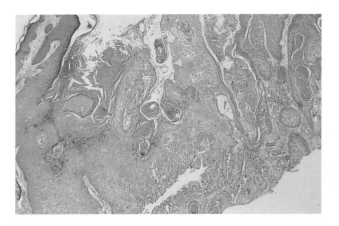

FIG. 22-89

Squamous cell carcinoma with the architecture of a keratoacanthoma. The lesion shows several horn-filled invaginations. On this low magnification the lesion looks like a keratoacanthoma. (× 10)

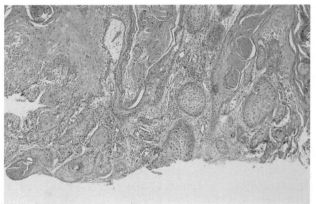

FIG. 22-90

Squamous cell carcinoma with the architecture of a keratoacanthoma. The base of the lesion consists of irregular lobules containing horn pearls. (× 16)

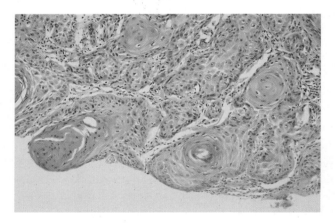

FIG. 22-91

Squamous cell carcinoma, higher magnification of Fig. 22-89. The base of the lesion consists of irregular tumor lobules containing horn pearls. Many of the nuclei are hyperchromatic. (× 40)

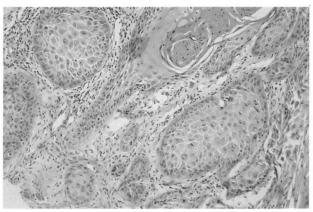

FIG. 22-92

Squamous cell carcinoma, higher magnification of Fig. 22-89. The base of the tumor consists of irregular lobules with atypical cells that vary in size. Several of the nuclei are hyperchromatic. (× 40)

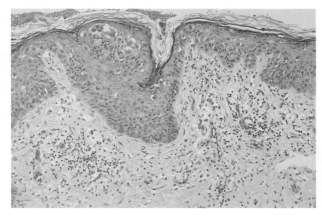

FIG. 22·93

Paget's disease of the nipple. Within the epidermis large rounded cells are seen that contain a large nucleus and ample cytoplasm. The cytoplasm of the Paget cells stains much lighter than the cytoplasm of the surroundings keratinocytes. (× 40)

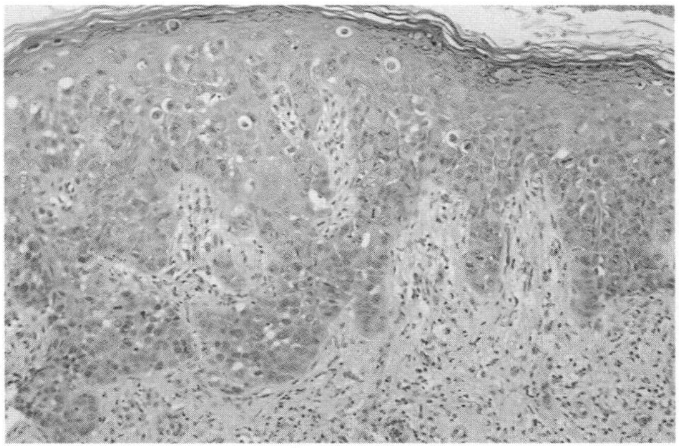

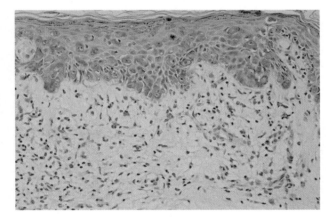

FIG. 22·94

Paget's disease of the nipple. Within the acanthotic epidermis large rounded cells with ample cystoplasm are seen. The cells do not form any intercellular bridges. The Paget cells lie singly and in small groups. (× 40)

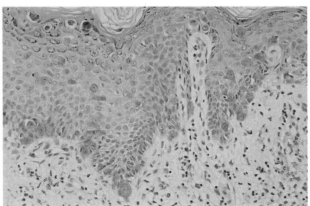

FIG. 22·95

Paget's disease of the nipple, incubated with a polyclonal antibody against carcinoembryonic antigen. The Paget cells show a positive reaction, the keratinocytes are negative. The Paget cells lie singly and in groups. ABC technique. (× 64)

FIG. 22·96

Paget's disease of the nipple, incubation with a polyclonal antibody against carcinoembryonic antigen (CEA). Within the acanthotic epidermis, scattered CEA-positive Paget cells are seen. ABC technique. (× 64)

C H A P T E R 23

Tumors of
the Epidermal
Appendages

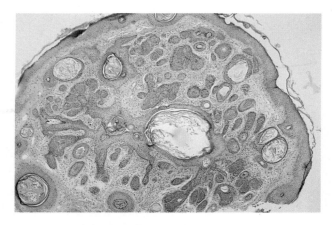

FIG. 23·1

Trichofolliculoma. The dermis contains a large cystic space that is lined by squamous epithelium and filled with keratin. Radiating from the wall of this "primary" hair follicle one sees many small, well-differentiated "secondary" hair follicles. (× 16)

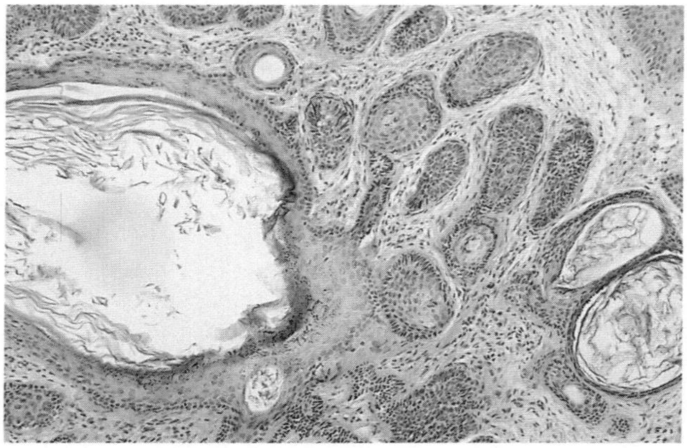

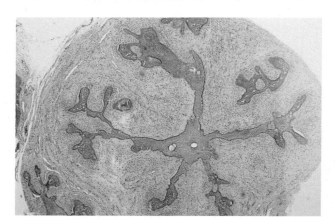

FIG. 23-2

Trichofolliculoma, higher magnification. Radiating from the horn-filled "primary" hair follicle are many small "secondary" hair follicles. The secondary hair follicles usually show an outer and inner root sheath. (× 40)

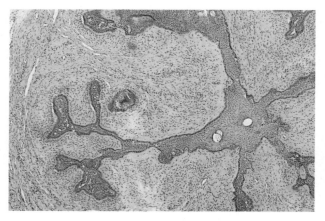

FIG. 23-3

Fibrofolliculoma. In the center of this photomicrograph a hair follicle is seen, from which thin bands of follicular epithelium extend into the stroma. The stroma stains basophilic and is mucoid. (× 10)

FIG. 23-4

Fibrofolliculoma. From a distorted hair follicle strands of follicular epithelium extend into a basophilic, mucoid stroma. (× 16)

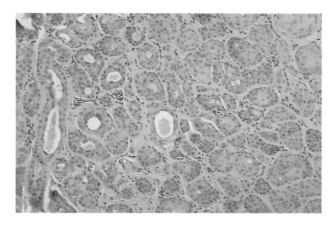

FIG. 23-5

Trichoepithelioma. The lesion contains several horn cysts, which are the most characteristic histologic feature. They consist of a fully keratinized center. The keratinization is abrupt and complete. (× 40)

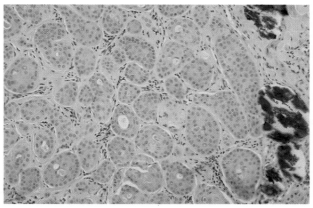

FIG. 23-6

Trichoepithelioma. The lesion shows several small horn cysts and calcium deposits, which stain dark red on H&E. (× 40)

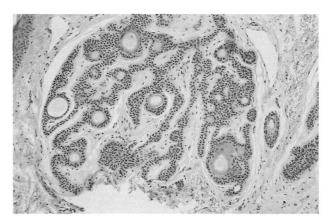

FIG. 23-7

Trichoepithelioma. The lesion shows strands of follicular epithelium containing several horn cysts. (× 40)

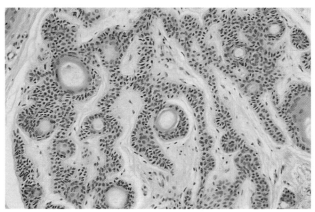

FIG. 23-8

Trichoepithelioma, higher magnification of Fig. 23-7. The horn cysts consist of a fully keratinized center. The keratinization is abrupt and complete. (× 64)

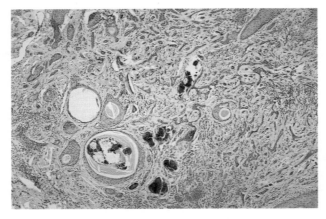

FIG. 23-9

Desmoplastic trichoepithelioma. The characteristic findings are (1) narrow strands of tumor cells, (2) horn cysts, and (3) a desmoplastic stroma. (× 16)

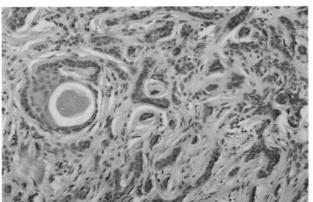

FIG. 23-10

Desmoplastic trichoepithelioma. The horn cyst has a fully keratinized center. The outer cell layer of the horn cyst stains basophilic, like in a basal cell epithelioma. Within the desmoplastic stroma innumerable thin strands of basophilic cells are seen. (× 64)

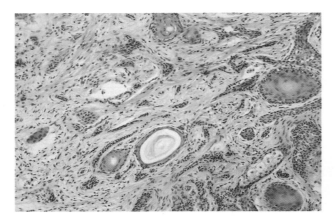

FIG. 23-11

Desmoplastic trichoepithelioma. The lesion shows horn cysts, thin strands of follicular epithelium, and a desmoplastic stroma. (× 40)

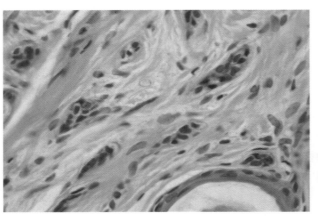

FIG. 23-12

Desmoplastic trichoepithelioma, higher magnification. Thin strands of basophilic tumor cells are seen in a densely collagenous and hypocellular stroma. (× 160)

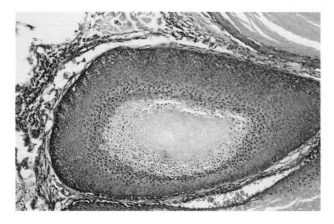

FIG. 23-13

Pilomatricoma (calcifying epithelioma). The tumor is sharply demarcated. Two types of cells are present: basophilic cells and shadow cells. This photomicrograph shows a gradual transition between basophilic cells and faintly eosinophilic, fully keratinized shadow cells. (× 40)

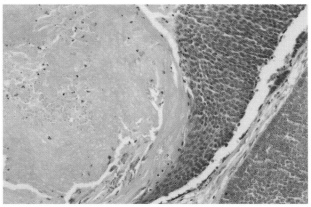

FIG. 23-14

Pilomatricoma (calcifying epithelioma). Higher magnification shows the two types of cells usually present in this lesion: basophilic cells and shadow cells. The shadow cells have a distinct border and possess a central unstained area as a shadow of the lost nucleus. (× 64)

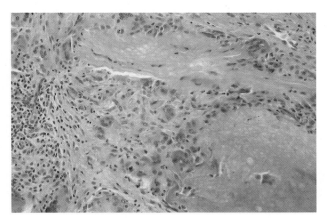

FIG. 23-15

Pilomatricoma (calcifying epithelioma). The stroma of the tumor usually shows a considerable foreign body giant cell reaction adjacent to the shadow cells. (× 64)

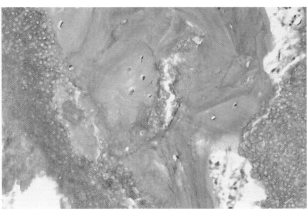

FIG. 23-16

Pilomatricoma (calcifying epithelioma). Occasionally foci of ossification are seen within a pilomatricoma. Ossification takes place in the stroma. (× 64)

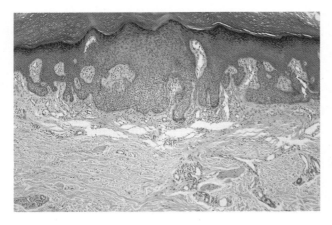

FIG. 23-17

Trichilemmoma. The tumor cells have the appearance of clear cells. The periphery of the tumor lobules shows palisading of columnar cells. (× 16)

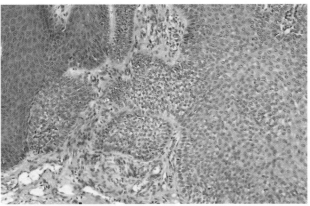

FIG. 23-18

Trichilemmoma, higher magnification. The tumor cells show a clear cytoplasm. At the periphery of the tumor lobule palisading of the basal cells is seen. (× 40)

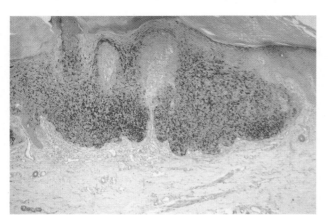

FIG. 23-19

Trichilemmoma, PAS stain. There is a rather sharp demarcation between PAS-positive tumor cells and PAS-negative normal keratinocytes. (× 16)

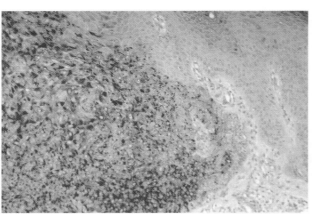

FIG. 23-20

Trichilemmoma, PAS stain. The clear cytoplasm of the tumor cells seen in H&E sections is due to accumulations of glycogen within the cells, which stains with the PAS reaction. (× 64)

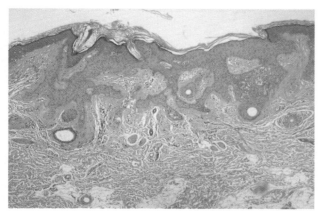

FIG. 23-21

Tumor of the follciular infundibulum. A platelike growth of pale-staining epithelial cells extends parallel to the epidermis in the upper dermis and shows multiple connections with the epidermis. (× 16)

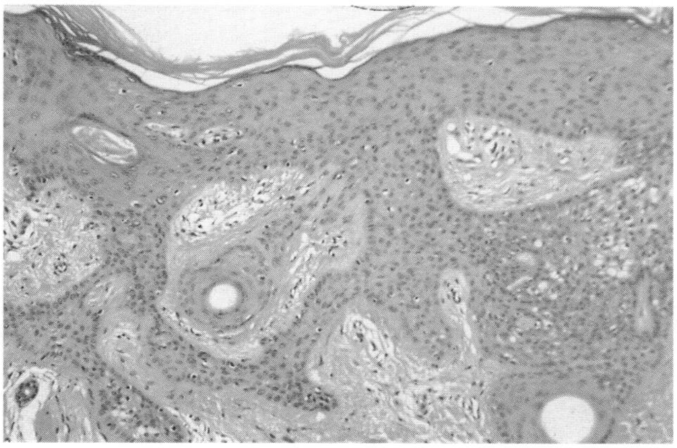

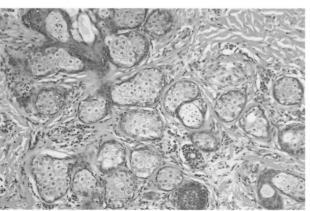

FIG. 23-22

Tumor of the follicular infundibulum. The peripheral cell layer of the tumor plate shows palisading, and the centrally located cells show a pale-staining cytoplasm as a result of their content of glycogen. (× 40)

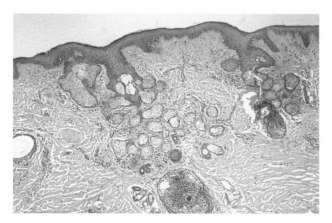

FIG. 23-23

Nevus sebaceus of a newborn. At birth numerous small sebaceous glands are seen in the corium. (× 16)

FIG. 23-24

Nevus sebaceus of a newborn. The sebaceous glands are numerous, but small. (× 40)

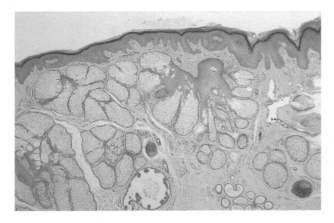

FIG. 23-25

Nevus sebaceus of an adult. Large numbers of mature sebaceous glands are present. Mature apocrine glands are located in the lower dermis. (× 10)

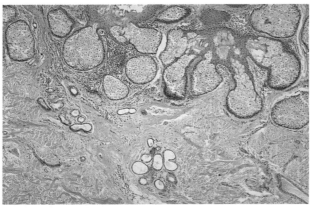

FIG. 23-26

Nevus sebaceus of an adult. Numerous mature sebaceous glands lie in the upper dermis. Ectopic apocrine glands are present in the lower dermis. (× 16)

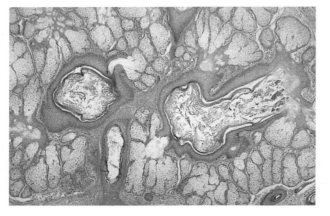

FIG. 23-27

Sebaceous hyperplasia. The lesion consists of a single greatly enlarged sebaceous gland composed of numerous lobules that are grouped around a centrally located, wide sebaceous duct. (× 16)

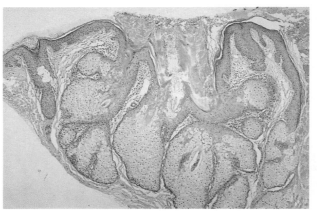

FIG. 23-28

Sebaceous hyperplasia. Around a centrally located, wide sebaceous duct, sebaceous lobules are grouped. (× 16)

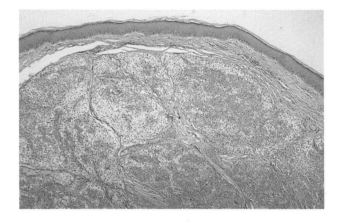

FIG. 23·29

Sebaceous adenoma. In the upper dermis a tumor consisting of sebaceous gland lobules can be seen. Germinative and sebaceous gland cells are present in approximately equal proportions. (× 16)

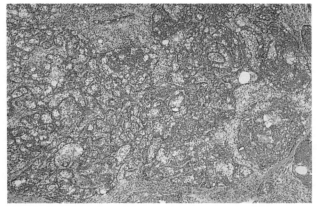

FIG. 23·30

Sebaceous adenoma. The tumor consists of sharply demarcated sebaceous lobules, which show incomplete differentiation. Two types of cells are present: undifferentiated basophilic germinative cells and mature sebaceous cells. (× 16)

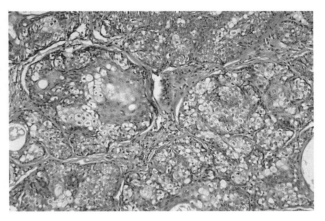

FIG. 23·31

Sebaceous adenoma. Sharply demarcated sebaceous lobules are present. Two types of cells are seen: germinative cells and mature sebaceous cells. Distribution of the two types of cells within the lobules varies. In most lobules the two types of cells occur in approximately equal proportions. (× 40)

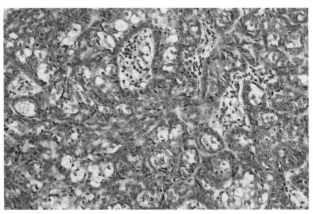

FIG. 23·32

Sebaceous adenoma. The germinative cells stain basophilic, the sebaceous cells have a pale cytoplasm, owing to accumulation of lipids. (× 64)

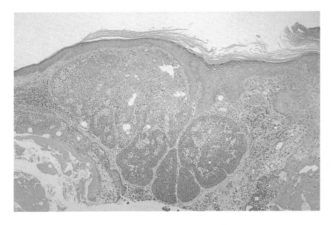

FIG. 23-33

Sebaceous epithelioma. Within the dermis a tumor consisting of sebaceous lobules is seen. The majority of cells are undifferentiated cells. (× 16)

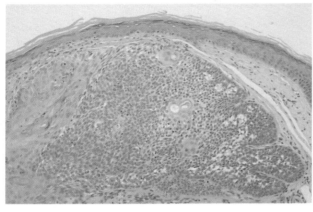

FIG. 23-34

Sebaceous epithelioma. Higher magnification shows that the majority of cells within a sebaceous lobule are germinative cells. (× 40)

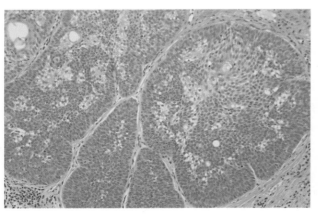

FIG. 23-35

Sebaceous epithelioma. The majority of cells are basophilic germinative cells. Groups of mature sebaceous cells lie in the center of most lobules. (× 40)

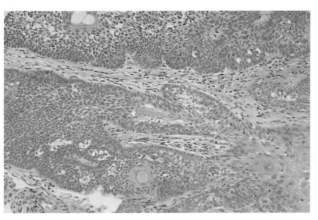

FIG. 23-36

Sebaceous epithelioma. The tumor grows in irregularly shaped masses. Within the tumor masses an occasional focus of keratinization may be visible. (× 40)

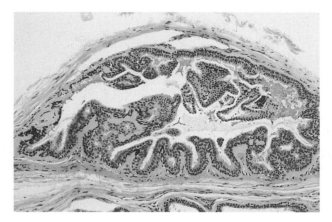

FIG. 23-37

Apocrine hidrocystoma. The dermis contains one large cystic space into which papillary projections extend. The luminal inner surface of the wall and the papillary projections are lined by a row of secretory cells showing "decapitation" secretion. (× 40)

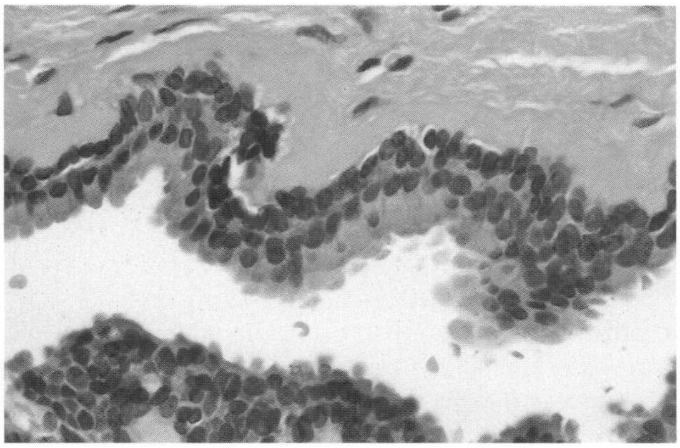

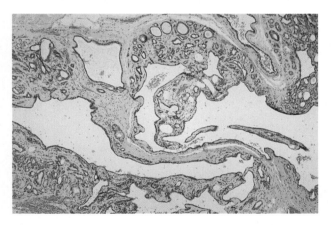

FIG. 23-38

Apocrine hidrocystoma, higher magnification showing apocrine secretion. Peripheral to the layer of secretory cells, myoepithelial cells can be seen. (× 160)

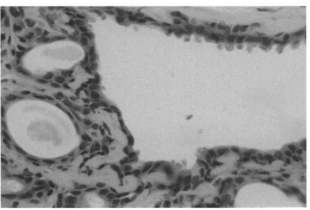

FIG. 23-39

Apocrine hidrocystoma. Several large cystic spaces are seen into which papillary projections extend. (× 16)

FIG. 23-40

Apocrine hidrocystoma, higher magnification showing evidence of "decapitation" secretion. (× 160)

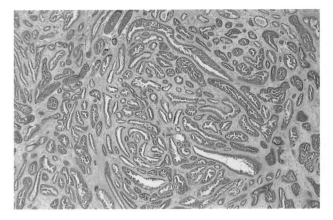

FIG. 23-41

Hidradenoma papilliferum. Within the tumor tubular and cystic structures are observed. They are lined by apocrine secretory cells. (× 10)

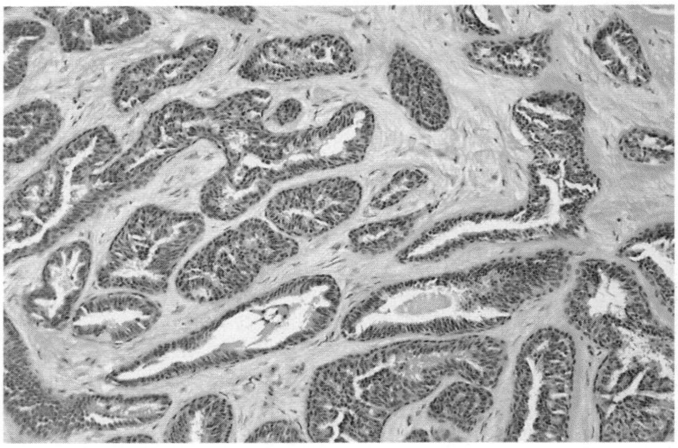

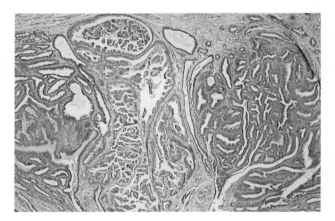

FIG. 23-42

Hidradenoma papilliferum. The tubular and cystic structures are lined by apocrine secretory cells. Peripheral to the apocrine secretory cells, myoepithelial cells are present. (× 40)

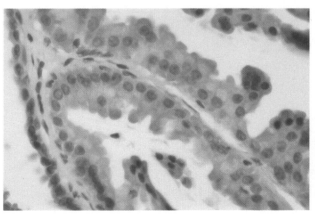

FIG. 23-43

Hidradenoma papilliferum. Tubular and cystic structures are seen. Papillary folds project into the cystic spaces. (× 16)

FIG. 23-44

Hidradenoma papilliferum, higher magnification. The lumina are lined by apocrine secretory cells, some of which show active decapitation secretion. Peripheral to the apocrine gland cells, elongated myoepithelial cells are present. (× 160)

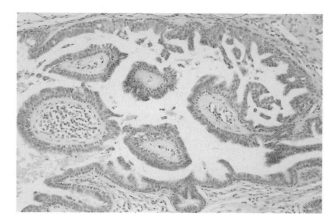

FIG. 23-45

Syringocystadenoma papilliferum. A cystic invagination extends down from the epidermis. Papillary projections extend into the lumina of the invagination. The papillary projections are lined by glandular epithelium and a row of myoepithelial cells. (× 40)

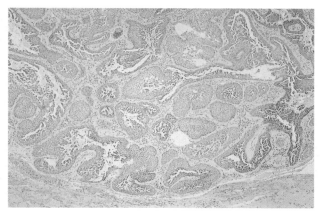

FIG. 23-46

Syringocystadenoma papilliferum. The papillary projections and the lower portion of the invaginations are lined by glandular epithelium. Some of the cells show active decapitation secretion. The stroma of the tumor contains numerous plasma cells. (× 40)

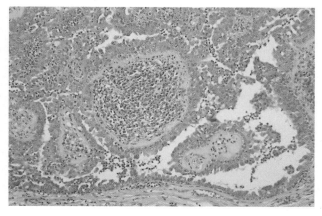

FIG. 23-47

Tubular apocrine adenoma. Numerous tubular structures are seen into which papillary projections extend. Cellular fragments are seen in several lumina. (× 16)

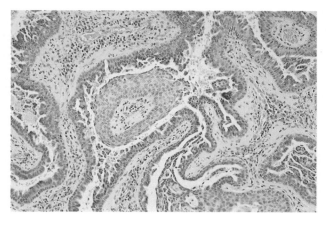

FIG. 23-48

Tubular apocrine adenoma. The papillary projections are lined by two rows of cells. The luminal row of cells consists of columnar cells that show apocrine secretion. The outer row of cells consists of small cuboidal cells. Decapitated portions of cells are seen in several lumina. (× 40)

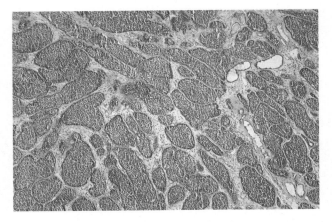

FIG. 23-49

Cylindroma. Numerous islands of epithelial cells are seen that lie close together. They seem to fit together like pieces of a jigsaw puzzle. (× 16)

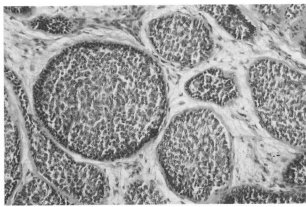

FIG. 23-50

Cylindroma, higher magnification. Two types of cells are present: cells with small, dark-staining nuclei are present at the periphery of the islands, often in a palisade arrangement. Cells with large, light-staining nuclei lie in the center of the islands. The tumor islands are surrounded by a hyalin sheath. (× 64)

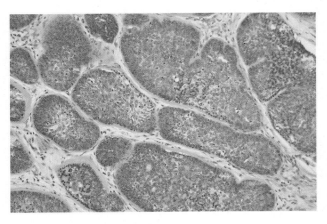

FIG. 23-51

Cylindroma. Each tumor island is surrounded by a hyalin sheath, which stains pink on H&E sections. (× 40)

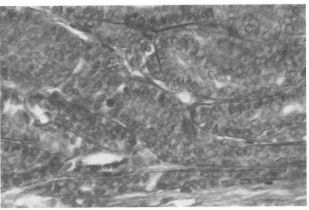

FIG. 23-52

Cylindroma, PAS stain. The hyalin sheath around each tumor lobule is PAS positive and diastase resistant. (× 160)

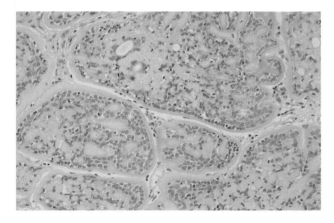

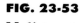
FIG. 23-53

Malignant cylindroma. The tumor islands show loss of palisading at the periphery. Some pleomorphism of nuclei can be seen. (× 64)

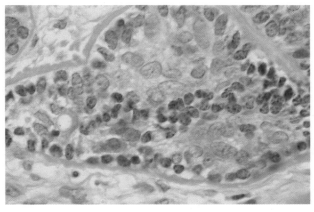

FIG. 23-54

Malignant cylindroma. The tumor island shows marked anaplasia and pleomorphism of the nuclei and loss of palisading at the periphery. (× 240)

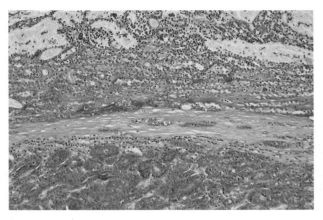

FIG. 23-55

Malignant cylindroma, PAS stain. The upper portion of the photomicrograph shows the malignant degeneration within the tumor; the lower portion shows parts of the benign cylindroma. Hyalin sheaths are partially lost around the malignant tumor islands. (× 40)

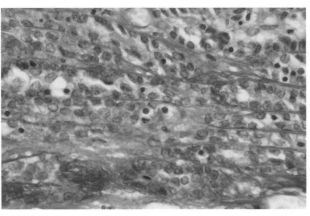

FIG. 23-56

Malignant cylindroma, PAS stain. The PAS-positive material is decreased. Several mitoses can be seen. There is no palisading at the periphery of each lobule. (× 160)

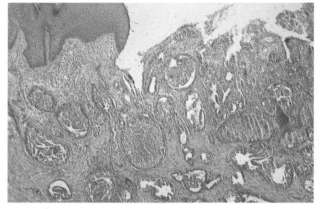

FIG. 23-57

Erosive adenomatosis of the nipple. Extending downward from the epidermis are irregular, dilated tubular structures. The tubules are lined by a peripheral layer of cuboidal cells and a luminal layer of columnar cells. (× 16)

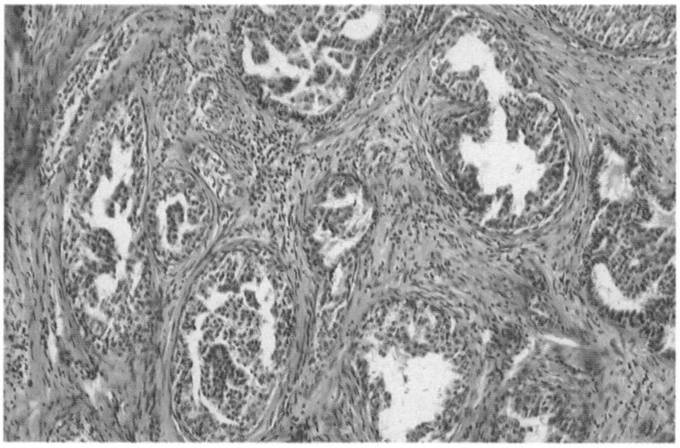

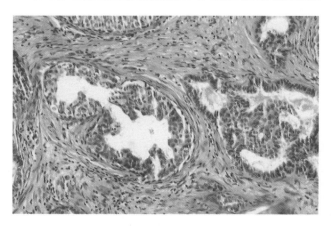

FIG. 23-58

Erosive adenomatosis of the nipple. The lumina contain partially necrotic cells. Several of the lumina contain papillary projections. (× 40)

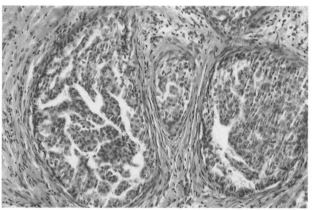

FIG. 23-59

Erosive adenomatosis of the nipple, higher magnification. The tubules are lined by a peripheral layer of cuboidal cells and a luminal layer of columnar cells. (× 64)

FIG. 23-60

Erosive adenomatosis of the nipple. The lumina contain groups of cells that are partially necrotic. (× 64)

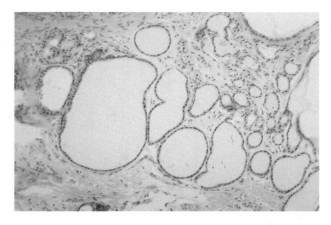

FIG. 23-61

Eccrine hidrocystoma. Several cystic lumina can be seen that are lined by flattened epithelium. (× 40)

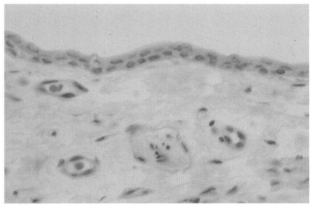

FIG. 23-62

Eccrine hidrocystoma, higher magnification of Fig. 23-61. The lumina are lined by two layers of small cuboidal cells. (× 160)

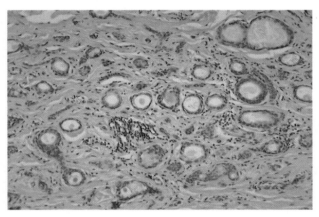

FIG. 23-63

Syringoma. Numerous small ducts are embedded in a fibrous stroma. The ducts are lined by two rows of epithelial cells. The lumina of the ducts contain amorphous debris. Some of the ducts possess small, commalike tails of epithelial cells, giving them the appearance of tadpoles. (× 40)

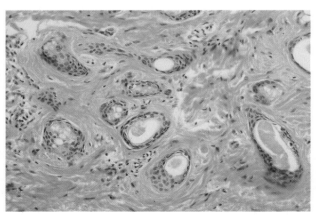

FIG. 23-64

Syringoma. The walls of the ducts are lined by two rows of epithelial cells. The lumina contain amorphous debris. (× 64)

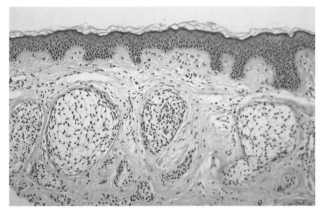

FIG. 23-65

Clear cell syringoma. Solid cell islands are predominantly seen. These islands are composed of clear cells. (× 40)

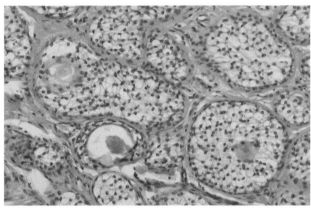

FIG. 23-66

Clear cell syringoma. The tumor islands are composed of clear cells. Several islands show small lumina. (× 64)

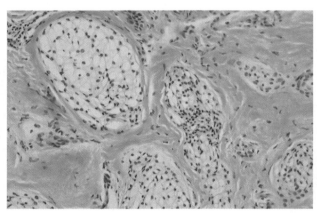

FIG. 23-67

Clear cell syringoma. The tumor islands are composed entirely of clear cells. (× 64)

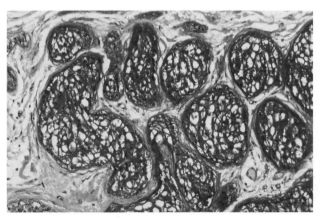

FIG. 23-68

Clear cell syringoma, PAS stain. The clear cytoplasm seen on H&E sections is due to accumulation of glycogen, which is PAS positive. (× 64)

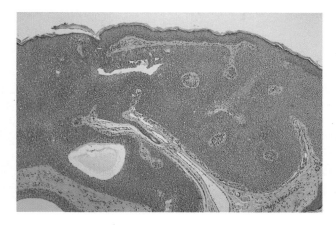

FIG. 23-69

Eccrine poroma. The tumor arises within the lower portion of the epidermis from where it extends downward into the dermis as tumor masses that consist of broad, anastomosing bands. (× 16)

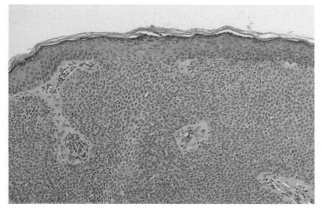

FIG. 23-70

Eccrine poroma. The border between epidermis and tumor is readily apparent because of the distinctive appearance of the tumor cells: they are smaller than squamous cells. (× 40)

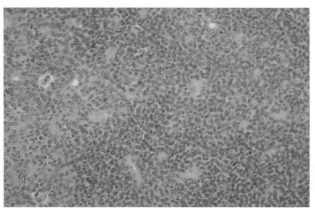

FIG. 23-71

Eccrine poroma. The tumor cells are smaller than squamous cells, have a uniform cuboidal appearance and a round, deeply basophilic nucleus. (× 64)

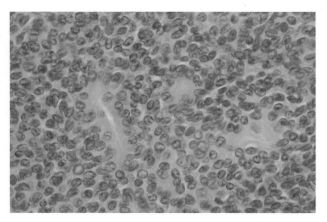

FIG. 23-72

Eccrine poroma. Narrow ductal lumina may be present within the tumor. They are lined by an eosinophilic, PAS-positive, diastase-resistant cuticle. (× 160)

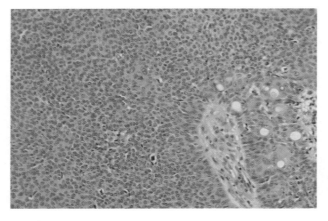

FIG. 23-73

Malignant eccrine poroma. Some of the tumor cells have hyperchromatic nuclei. (× 40)

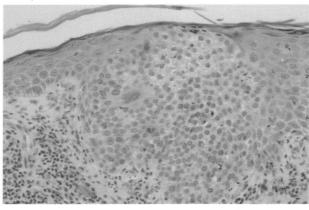

FIG. 23-74

Malignant eccrine poroma. Some of the tumor cells have a pale cytoplasm because of the accumulation of glycogen. (× 64)

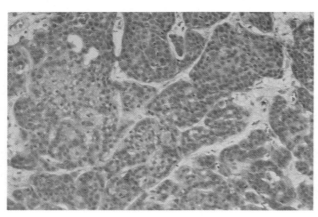

FIG. 23-75

Malignant eccrine poroma. The tumor consists of irregularly shaped lobules with pleomorphic nuclei. (× 40)

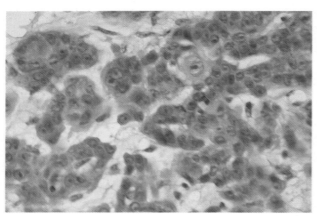

FIG. 23-76

Malignant eccrine poroma, higher magnification. The malignant cells have large, hyperchromatic, irregularly shaped nuclei. They have a pale-staining cytoplasm because of the accumulation of glycogen. (× 160)

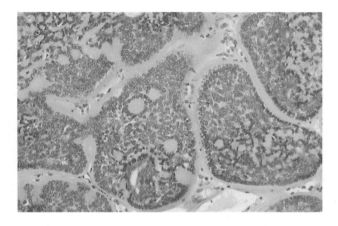

FIG. 23-77

Eccrine spiradenoma. One large tumor lobule is located within the dermis. The tumor lobule appears deeply basophilic because of the close aggregation of nuclei. Several lumina are present. (× 40)

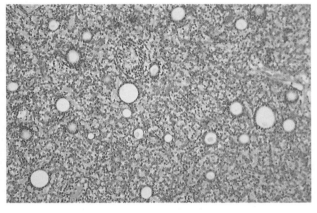

FIG. 23-78

Eccrine spiradenoma. The tumor usually consists of several sharply demarcated lobules. The tumor islands enclose small islands of connective tissue. (× 64)

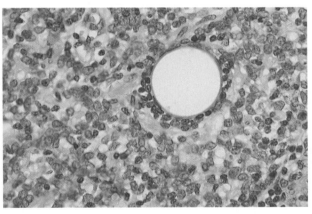

FIG. 23-79

Eccrine spiradenoma. The tumor island consists of intertwining cords of two types of cells. The cells of the first type possess small, dark nuclei. The cells of the second type have large, pale nuclei. (× 160)

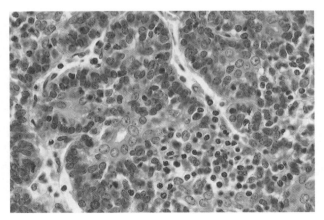

FIG. 23-80

Eccrine spiradenoma. The cells with the dark nuclei are usually located at the periphery of the lobule, whereas the cells with the large, pale nuclei are located in the center of the lobules. (× 160)

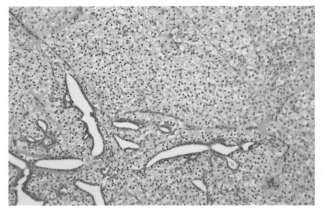

FIG. 23-81

Clear cell hidradenoma. Within the lobular masses tubular lumina of various sizes are present. The tubular lumina are lined by cuboidal ductal cells. (× 40)

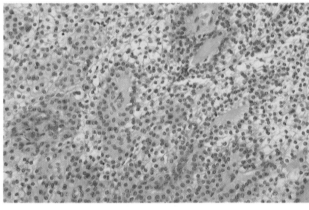

FIG. 23-82

Clear cell hidradenoma. The cells have a clear cytoplasm. (× 64)

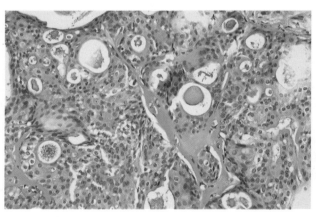

FIG. 23-83

Clear cell hidradenoma. Numerous cystic spaces are seen that contain faintly eosinophilic, homogeneous material. (× 64)

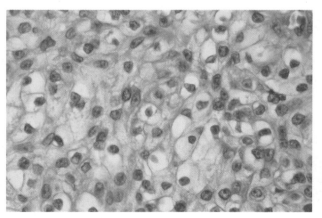

FIG. 23-84

Clear cell hidradenoma. The cells have a clear cytoplasm with dark nuclei. (× 160)

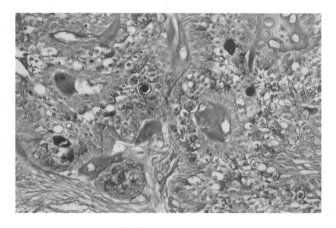

FIG. 23-85

Clear cell hidradenoma, PAS stain. The tumor cells and the amorphous material within the cystic spaces are PAS positive. (× 64)

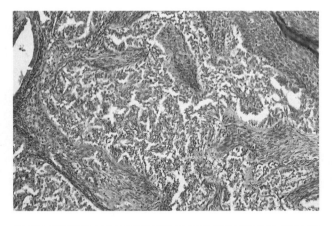

FIG. 23-86

Clear cell hidradenoma. Most of the tumor cells contain considerable amounts of glycogen, which is PAS positive. (× 64)

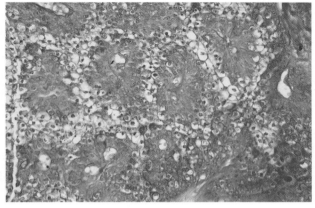

FIG. 23-87

Malignant clear cell hidradenoma. The tumor islands show invasion into the surrounding tissue. (× 40)

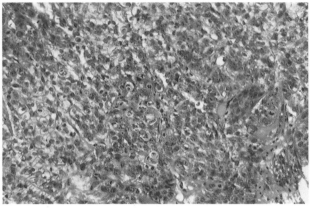

FIG. 23-88

Malignant clear cell hidradenoma. The tumor cells show nuclear anaplasia and hyperchromatic nuclei. (× 64)

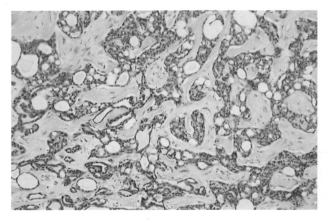

FIG. 23-89

Chondroid syringoma. Tubular and cystic, partially branching lumina can be seen. The lumina are embedded in an abundant stroma. (× 40)

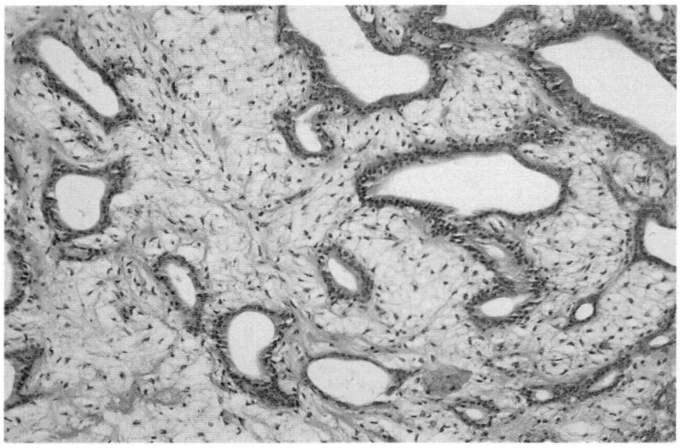

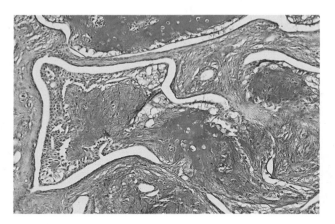

FIG. 23-90

Chondroid syringoma. The tubular lumina are lined by two layers of epithelial cells: a luminal layer of cuboidal cells and a peripheral layer of flattened cells. The stroma is pale. (× 40)

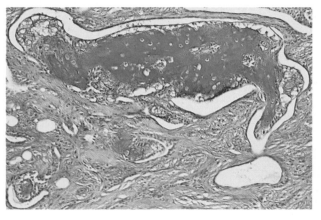

FIG. 23-91

Chondroid syringoma, alcian stain. The stroma stains positively because of the presence of sulfated acid mucopolysaccharides, that is, chondroitin sulfate. (× 40)

FIG. 23-92

Chondroid syringoma, alcian stain. The stroma stains blue. (× 40)

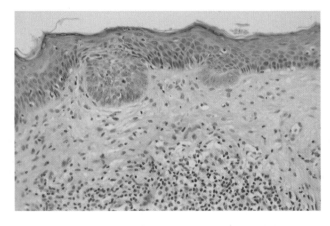

FIG. 23-93

Superficial basal cell epithelioma. Buds are seen attached to the undersurface of the epidermis. (× 64)

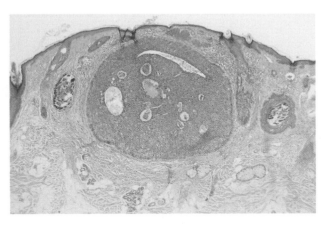

FIG. 23-94

Superficial basal cell epithelioma. The peripheral cell layer of the tumor formation shows palisading. The overlying epidermis is slightly atrophic. Fibroblasts are arranged around the tumor cell proliferations. (× 64)

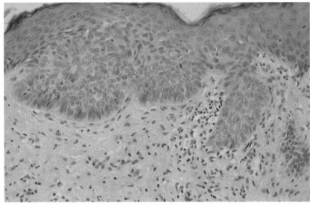

FIG. 23-95

Solid basal cell epithelioma. A well-demarcated tumor island is seen in the dermis. Within the stroma an area of calcification can be seen. (× 10)

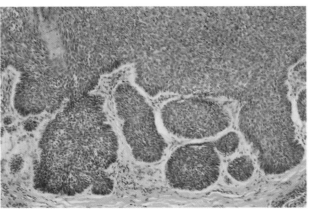

FIG. 23-96

Solid basal cell epithelioma. The peripheral cell layer of the tumor masses shows a palisade arrangement, whereas the nuclei inside the tumor masses lie in a haphazard fashion. (× 40)

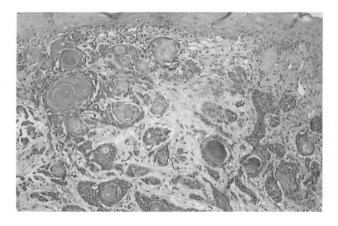

FIG. 23·97

Keratotic basal cell epithelioma. In addition to undifferentiated cells, there are parakeratotic cells and horn cysts. The parakeratotic cells have an eosinophilic cytoplasm. They lie in strands, in concentric whorls, or around the horn cysts. (× 40)

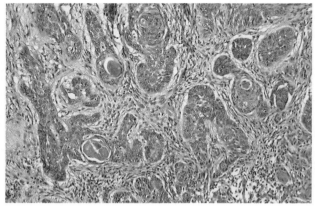

FIG. 23·98

Keratotic basal cell epithelioma. The tumor strands show several small horn cysts. (× 40)

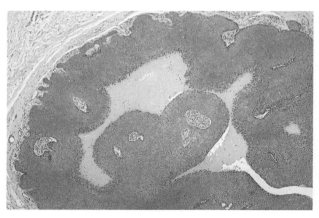

FIG. 23·99

Cystic basal cell epithelioma. Within the tumor lobules cystic spaces are seen. The cysts form as a result of necrobiotic changes in the centrally located tumor cells. (× 16)

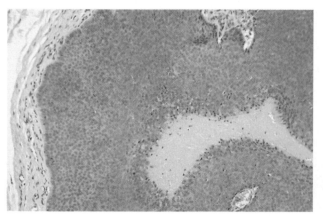

FIG. 23·100

Cystic basal cell epithelioma. The tumor lobule shows a palisade arrangement of the peripheral row of basal cells. (× 64)

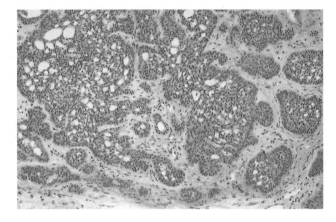

FIG. 23·101

Adenoid basal cell epithelioma. Formations are seen that suggest tubular, glandlike structures. The strands of epithelial cells present a lacelike pattern. (× 40)

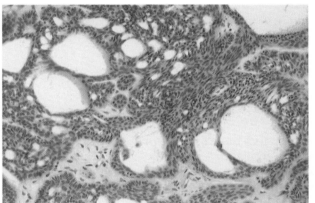

FIG. 23·102

Adenoid basal cell epithelioma. The tumor islands contain lumina that are partially lined by columnar cells. Several lumina contain granular material. (× 64)

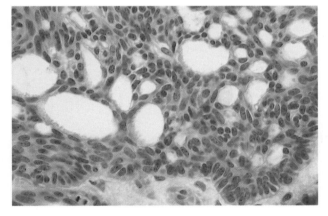

FIG. 23·103

Adenoid basal cell epithelioma. The lacelike pattern of the tumor is apparent. The tumor contains lumina surrounded by cells that have the appearance of glandular cells. (× 160)

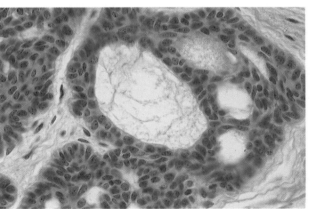

FIG. 23·104

Adenoid basal cell epithelioma. The lumina contain a granular material. (× 160)

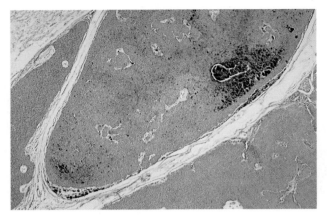

FIG. 23-105

Pigmented basal cell epithelioma. The large amounts of melanin seen in this lesion are mainly present in melanocytes and their dendrites, rather than in keratinocytes. (× 16)

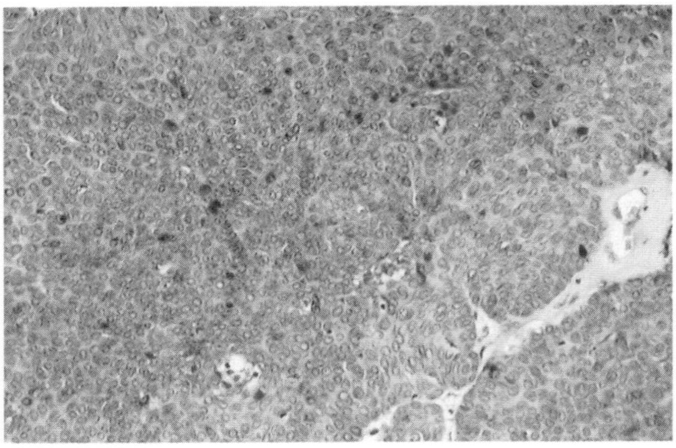

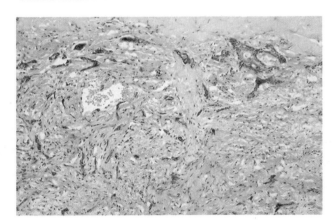

FIG. 23-106

Pigmented basal cell epithelioma. Heavily pigmented melanocytes are interspersed between keratinocytes. The melanin stays mostly in melanocytes because the tumor cells are unable to accept more than a small amount of melanin. (× 64)

FIG. 23-107

Fibrosing basal cell epithelioma. Embedded in a dense fibrous stroma are innumerable groups of tumor cells arranged in elongated strands. Most of the strands are narrow. (× 40)

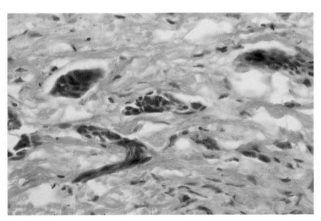

FIG. 23-108

Fibrosing basal cell epithelioma. Most of the strands are narrow and embedded in a dense fibrous stroma. (× 160)

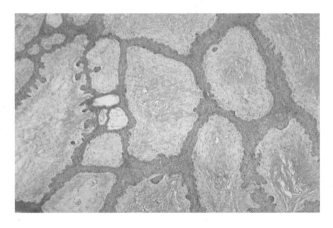

FIG. 23-109

Fibroepithelioma. Long, thin, branching, anastomosing strands of basal cell epithelioma are embedded in a fibrous stroma. (× 16)

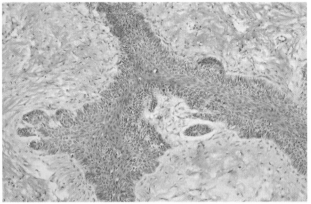

FIG. 23-110

Fibroepithelioma. Small groups of dark-staining cells showing a palisade arrangement of the peripheral cell layer may be seen along the epithelial strands. (× 40)

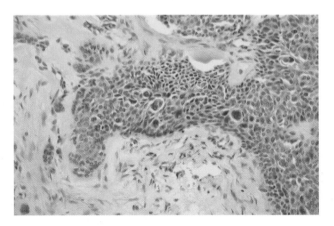

FIG. 23-111

Basal cell epithelioma with large nuclei. Within this area of basal cell epithelioma, several large atypical nuclei are seen. (× 64)

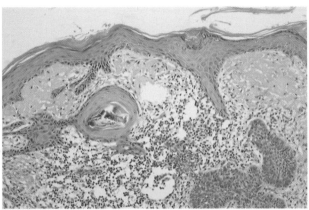

FIG. 23-112

Mixed carcinoma (basal cell epithelioma and squamous cell carcinoma). A squamous cell carcinoma (left) and a basal cell carcinoma lie side by side. (× 64)

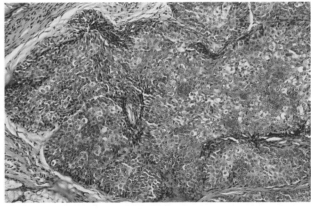

FIG. 23-113

Sebaceous gland carcinoma. The tumor shows irregular formations. The tumor lobules consist of undifferentiated and sebaceous cells. (× 40)

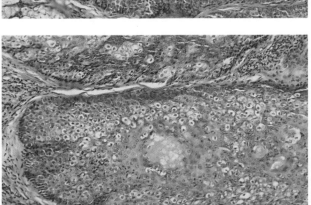

FIG. 23-114

Sebaceous gland carcinoma. Many of the undifferentiated cells have an eosinophilic cytoplasm. This lobule shows an area composed of atypical keratinizing cells. (× 40)

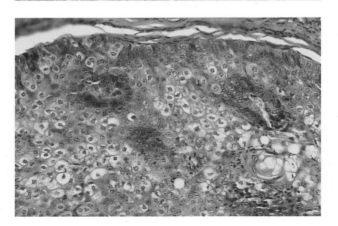

FIG. 23-115

Sebaceous gland carcinoma. The tumor consists of undifferentiated and sebaceous cells. Many of the undifferentiated cells have an eosinophilic cytoplasm. On the right side an area of atypical keratinization is seen. (× 64)

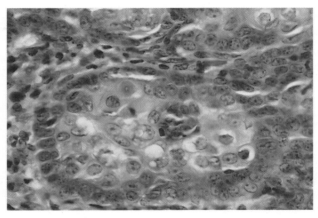

FIG. 23-116

Sebaceous gland carcinoma. The atypical cells show variation in size and shape of their nuclei. (× 160)

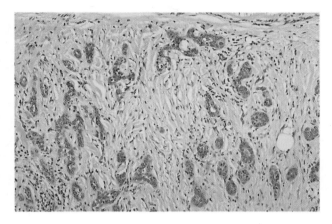

FIG. 23·117

Carcinoma of eccrine sweat glands. The tumor consists of largely tubular structures. Some of the tubules show a narrow lumen. (× 40)

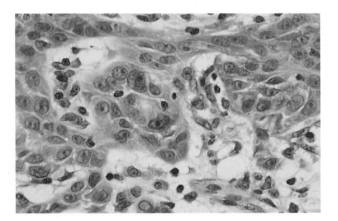

FIG. 23·118

Carcinoma of eccrine sweat glands. The tubular structures have only narrow lumina lined by a single layer or a double layer of cells. (× 64)

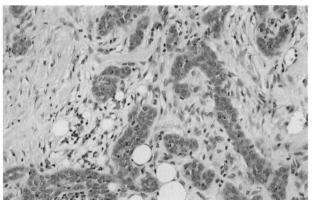

FIG. 23·119

Carcinoma of eccrine sweat glands. The tumor cells show considerable variation in size and shape of their nuclei. (× 160)

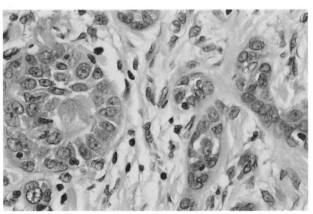

FIG. 23·120

Carcinoma of eccrine sweat glands. The tubular structures show only small lumina that may be lined by an eosinophilic cuticle. (× 160)

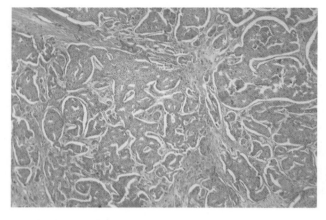

FIG. 23-121

Carcinoma of apocrine glands. Well-developed glandular lumina are present. The lumina may show branching. (× 16)

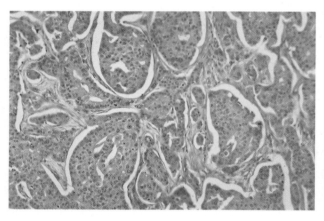

FIG. 23-122

Carcinoma of apocrine glands. The cytoplasm of the tumor cells is eosinophilic. Well-developed glandular lumina are present. (× 40)

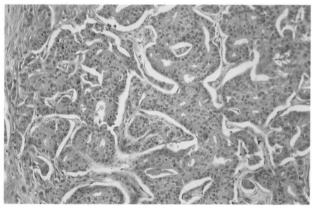

FIG. 23-123

Carcinoma of apocrine glands. The tumor consists of atypical glandular cells with eosinophilic cytoplasm and active "decapitation" secretion. (× 40)

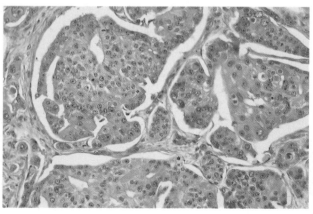

FIG. 23-124

Carcinoma of apocrine glands. The tumor cells show moderate nuclear anaplasia and an eosinophilic cytoplasm. (× 64)

CHAPTER 24

Metastatic Carcinoma

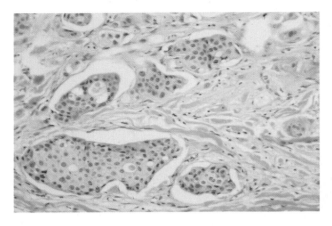

FIG. 24-1

Cutaneous metastasis from carcinoma of the breast, inflammatory carcinoma. The dermal lymphatics are filled with clusters of tumor cells. (× 40)

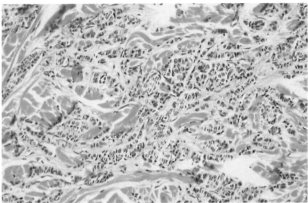

FIG. 24-2

Cutaneous metastasis from carcinoma of the breast, nodular carcinoma. Groups of tumor cells are surrounded by fibrotic collagen. (× 40)

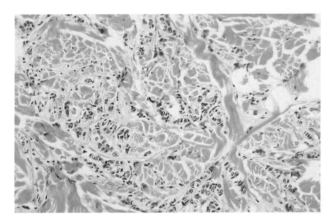

FIG. 24-3

Cutaneous metastasis from carcinoma of the breast, nodular carcinoma. Small groups of tumor cells in the dermis are surrounded by fibrosis. (× 40)

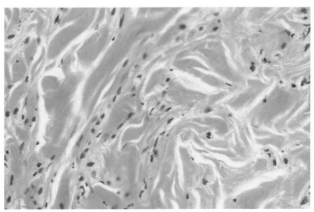

FIG. 24-4

Cutaneous metastatis from carcinoma of the breast, cancer en cuirasse. The indurated areas show fibrosis and only a few tumor cells, which may easily be overlooked because of their resemblance to fibroblasts. The tumor cells often lie singly, in small groups or in single-row lines, between thickened collagen bundles. (× 64)

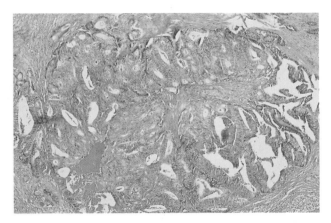

FIG. 24-5

Cutaneous metastasis from carcinoma of the colon. The metastasis consists of lobules with lumina. The lumina are lined with columnar cells. (× 16)

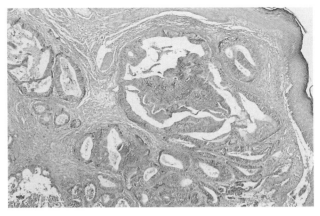

FIG. 24-6

Cutaneous metastasis from carcinoma of the colon. The lumina are lined by columnar cells and often contain groups of anaplastic cells. (× 16)

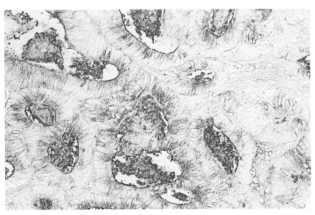

FIG. 24-7

Cutaneous metastasis from carcinoma of the colon, incubation with a polyclonal antibody against carcinoembryonic antigen. The tumor cells show a positive reaction (orange color). PAP technique. (× 40)

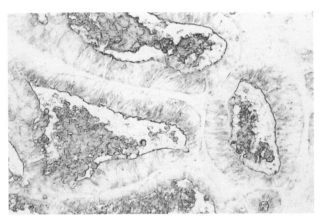

FIG. 24-8

Cutaneous metastasis from carcinoma of the colon. When incubated with a polyclonal antibody against carcinoembryonic antigen, the apical portion of the columnar cells lining the lumina show a positive reaction. In addition, the cellular debris within the lumina stains positively. (× 64)

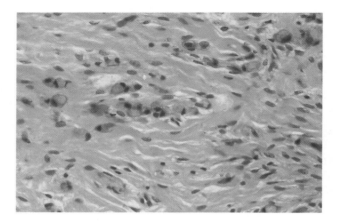

FIG. 24-9

Cutaneous metastasis from carcinoma of the stomach. Within the dermis irregularly grouped cells are present. They are large, round cells filled with mucin, which presses the nucleus against the cell wall. These cells are called signet-ring cells. (× 64)

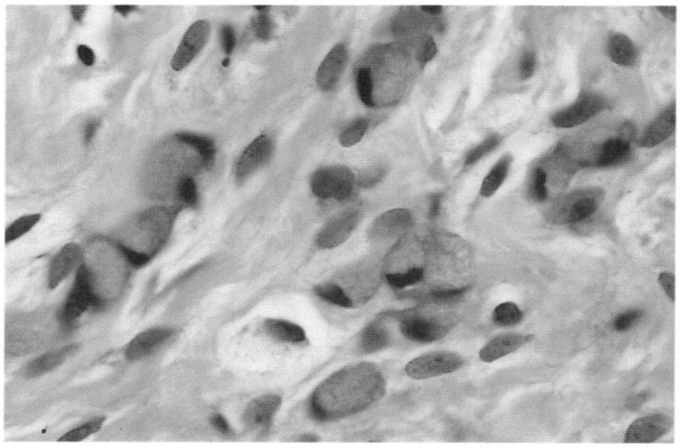

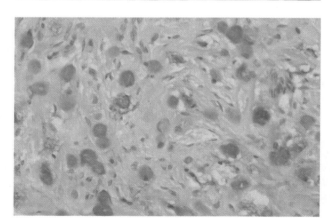

FIG. 24-10

Cutaneous metastasis from carcinoma of the stomach. The signet-ring cells are large, round cells filled with mucin, which presses the nucleus against the cell wall. The mucin is of the sialomucin type. (× 240)

FIG. 24-11

Cutaneous metastasis from carcinoma of the stomach, alcian stain. The mucin in the signet-ring cells stains blue with alcian at pH 2.5. (× 64)

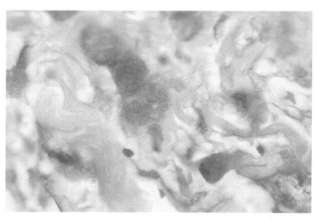

FIG. 24-12

Cutaneous metastasis from carcinoma of the stomach. The mucin within the signet-ring cells stains blue with alcian at pH 2.5 but not at pH 0.4, indicating that the acid mucopolysaccharides in the sialomucin are nonsulfated. (× 240)

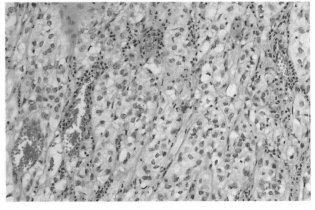

FIG. 24-13

Cutaneous metastasis from carcinoma of the kidney. The metastasis consists of large, polyhedral cells arranged in tubular, glandlike structures. The stroma of the metastasis is richly vascular, leading to extravasation of erythrocytes. (× 40)

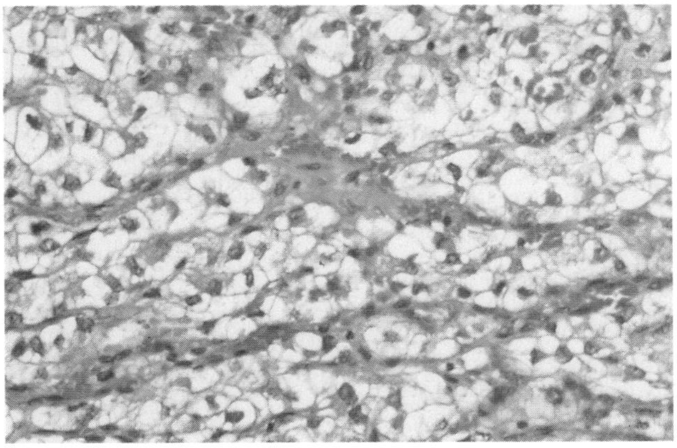

FIG. 24-14

Cutaneous metastasis from carcinoma of the kidney. The tumor cells have light-staining, centrally located nuclei and abundant, pale cytoplasm. The pale appearance of the cytoplasm is due to the presence of glycogen. Extravasation of erythrocytes into the glandlike structures is seen. (× 64)

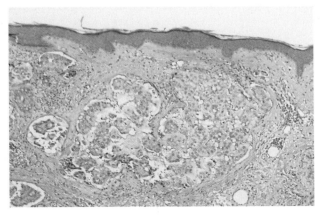

FIG. 24-15

Cutaneous metastasis from an adenocarcinoma of a bronchus. Within the dermis a metastasis composed of glandular structures with formation of mucin can be seen. (× 16)

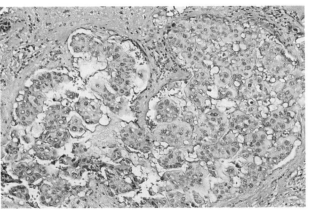

FIG. 24-16

Cutaneous metastasis from an adenocarcinoma of a bronchus. The atypical glandular structures show evidence of mucin formation. (× 40)

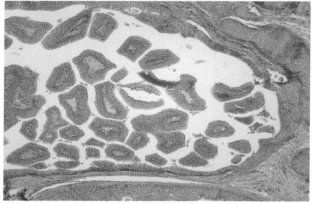

FIG. 24-17

Cutaneous metastasis from a papillary transitional cell carcinoma of the bladder. The metastatic lesion shows papillary growth. Each papilla is covered with transitional epithelium. (× 16)

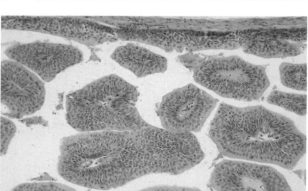

FIG. 24-18

Cutaneous metastasis from a papillary transitional cell carcinoma of the bladder, higher magnification of Fig. 24-17. The papillae are covered with transitional epithelium. (× 40)

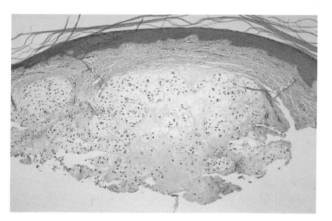

FIG. 24-19

Cutaneous metastasis from a chondrosarcoma. A well-circumscribed nodular lesion consisting of malignant chondrocytes is seen. (× 16)

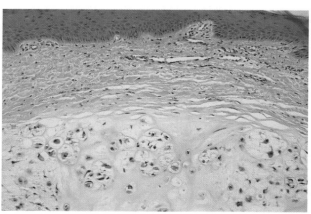

FIG. 24-20

Cutaneous metastasis from a chondrosarcoma. The lesion is characterized by hypercellularity, increase in nuclear size, and several cells with plump, multiple nuclei. (× 40)

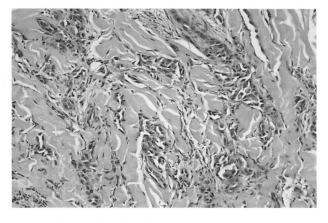

FIG. 24-21

Cutaneous metastasis from carcinoma of the prostate. Strands of tumor cells are seen in the dermis. (× 40)

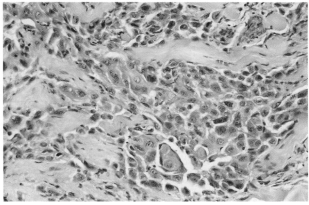

FIG. 24-22

Cutaneous metastasis from carcinoma of the prostate. The tumor islands consist of cuboidal cells with distinct cellular borders. (× 64)

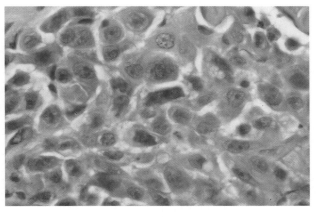

FIG. 24-23

Cutaneous metastasis from carcinoma of the prostate. The tumor cells are polygonal with small, round, hyperchromatic nuclei and scant cytoplasm. (× 160)

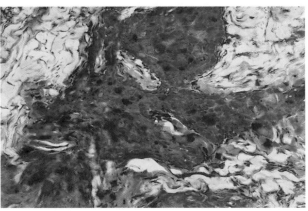

FIG. 24-24

Cutaneous metastasis from carcinoma of the prostate. Acid phosphatase (red reduction product) is present in the tumor cells. (× 64)

CHAPTER 25

Tumors of
Fibrous Tissue

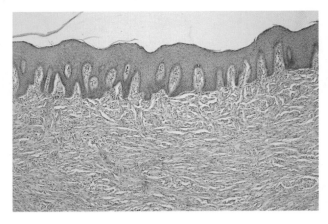

FIG. 25-1

Dermatofibroma, fibrous type. The epidermis is hyperplastic. Within the dermis intertwining collagen bundles are seen. (× 16)

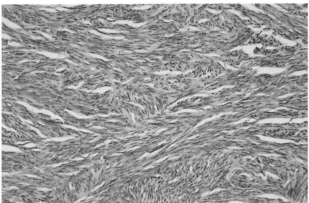

FIG. 25-2

Dermatofibroma, fibrous type. The collagen is irregularly arranged in intertwining and anastomosing bands, a so-called storiform (matlike) pattern. (× 40)

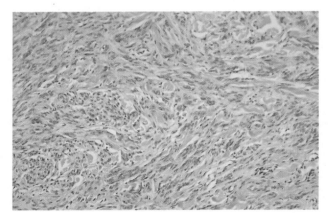

FIG. 25-3

Dermatofibroma, fibrous type, edge of the lesion. The dermatofibroma shows poor lateral demarcation, so that the fibroblasts and the young basophilic collagen of the tumor extend between the mature, eosinophilic collagen bundles of the dermis and surround them, thus trapping normal collagen bundles at the periphery of the nodule. (× 40)

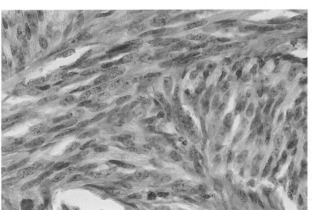

FIG. 25-4

Dermatofibroma, higher magnification of Fig. 25-2. The nuclei of the fibroblasts are elongated, and the fibroblasts have hardly any cytoplasm. They seem to radiate from a central point or "hub" in a whorllike fashion, giving them the appearance of a cartwheel. (× 160)

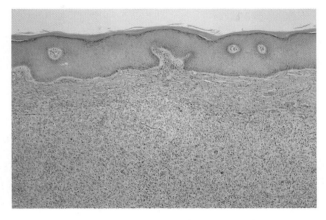

FIG. 25-5

Dermatofibroma, cellular type. The epidermis is hyperplastic. The tumor in the dermis is separated from the epidermis by a narrow band of almost normal collagen. (× 16)

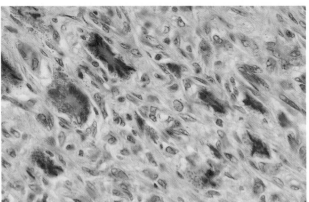

FIG. 25-6

Dermatofibroma, cellular type. The tumor consists of many cells with round to oval nuclei and ample cytoplasm. Several giant cells are present that contain phagocytized hemosiderin. (× 160)

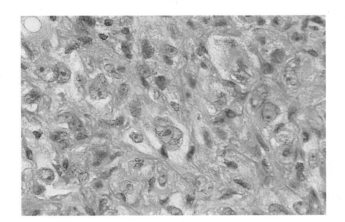

FIG. 25-7

Dermatofibroma, cellular type. Within the tumor numerous foam cells are seen with a vacuolated cytoplasm. They contain lipid. (× 160)

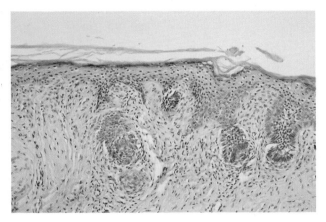

FIG. 25-8

Dermatofibroma. The epidermis overlying a dermatofibroma is hyperplastic and shows budding proliferations resembling a superficial basal cell epithelioma. (× 40)

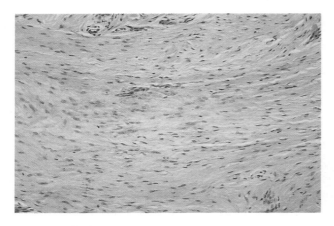

FIG. 25-9

Scar. The collagen fibers with fibroblasts are arranged in rows parallel to the epidermis. (× 40)

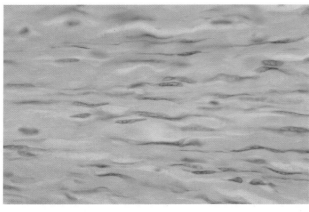

FIG. 25-10

Scar, higher magnification. The fibroblasts have long narrow nuclei. The collagen fibers show a parallel, wavy orientation. (× 160)

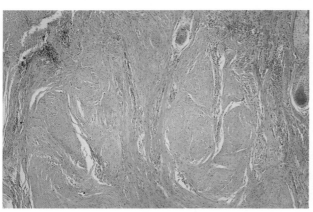

FIG. 25-11

Keloid. The collagen bundles are arranged in a whorllike or nodular pattern. (× 16)

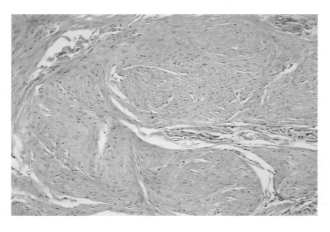

FIG. 25-12

Keloid. The nodules show thick, highly compacted, hyalinized bands of collagen lying in a concentric arrangement. (× 40)

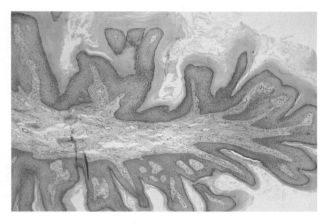

FIG. 25-13

Acrochordon. The lesion shows papillomatosis, hyperkeratosis, and regular acanthosis. (× 16)

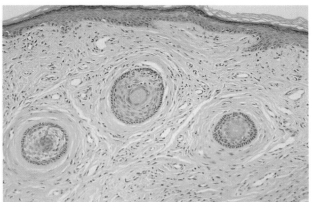

FIG. 25-14

Perifollicular fibroma. The hair follicles are surrounded by concentrically arranged young collagen. (× 16)

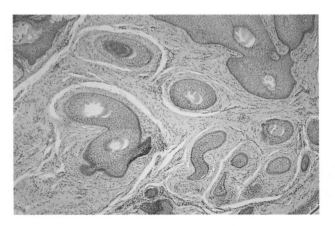

FIG. 25-15

Perifollicular fibroma. Concentric layers of collagen surround the hair follicles. The hair follicles are dilated. (× 16)

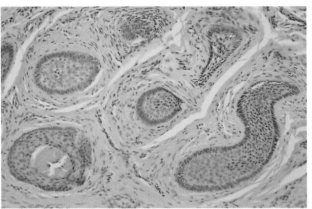

FIG. 25-16

Perifollicular fibroma, higher magnification. A hair follicle is dilated in the left lower corner and contains keratinous material. The follicles are surrounded by concentrically arranged young collagen showing numerous spindle-shaped nuclei. (× 40)

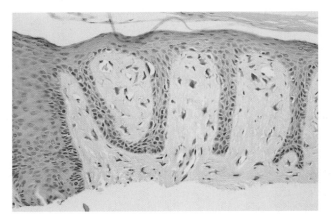

FIG. 25-17

Fibrous papule of the face (nose). The epidermis shows elongation of the rete ridges, hyperplastic melanocytes, and stellate fibroblasts. (× 64)

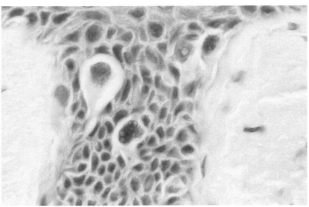

FIG. 25-18

Fibrous papule of the face (nose). The melanocytes in the epidermis are increased in size. (× 240)

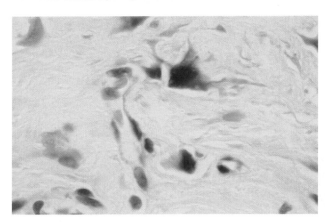

FIG. 25-19

Fibrous papule of the face (nose). The fibroblasts are plump, spindle-shaped, stellate. (× 240)

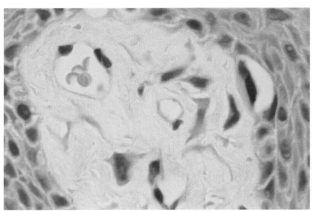

FIG. 25-20

Fibrous papule of the face (nose). Spindle-shaped, plump, stellate fibroblasts are present in the dermis. The melanocytes in the basal layer are increased in number and size. (× 240)

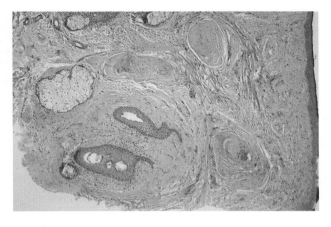

FIG. 25-21

Tuberous sclerosis. The main findings are dermal fibrosis and dilatation of some of the capillaries. (× 16)

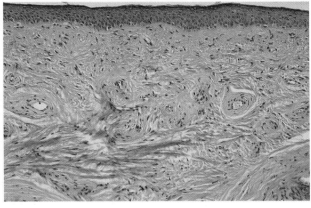

FIG. 25-22

Tuberous sclerosis. Concentric layers of thickened collagen are seen around capillaries. (× 40)

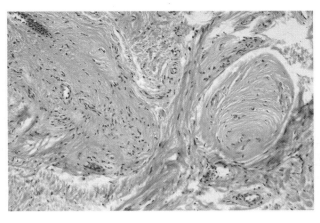

FIG. 25-23

Tuberous sclerosis. Perifollicular proliferation of collagen has led to compression of atrophic hair follicles by concentric layers of collagen. (× 64)

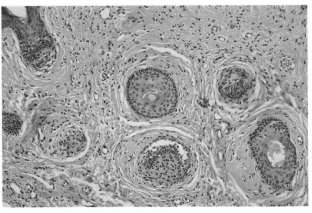

FIG. 25-24

Tuberous sclerosis. Sclerotic collagen is arranged in thick, concentric layers around atrophic pilosebaceous follicles. (× 40)

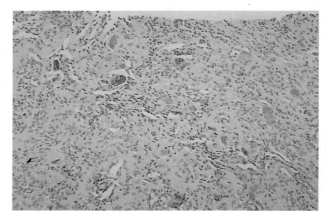

FIG. 25-25

Giant cell tumor of the tendon sheath. Numerous large, irregularly shaped, multinucleated giant cells are present. Most other cells have the appearance of fibroblasts. (× 40)

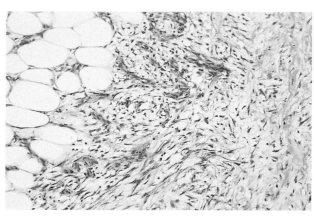

FIG. 25-26

Giant cell tumor of the tendon sheath. The giant cells have a deeply eosinophilic cytoplasm and contain a variable number of haphazardly distributed nuclei. (× 160)

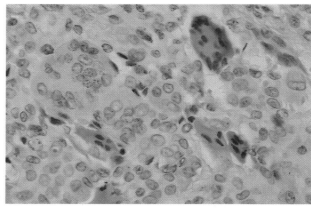

FIG. 25-27

Nodular pseudosarcomatous fasciitis. Numerous large pleomorphic fibroblasts are present that grow haphazardly in a stroma that contains varying amounts of mucinous ground substance. (× 40)

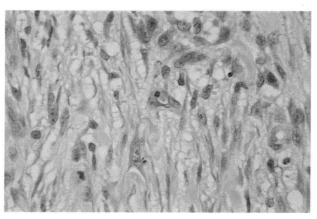

FIG. 25-28

Nodular pseudosarcomatous fasciitis. Numerous large, pleomorphic fibroblasts grow haphazardly in a mucinous stroma. (× 160)

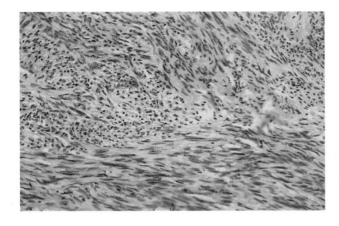

FIG. 25-29

Dermatofibrosarcoma protuberans. The tumor is composed predominantly of cells with large, spindle-shaped nuclei embedded in varying amounts of collagen. The nuclei are closely spaced and show pleomorphism and a moderate degree of atypicality. (× 64)

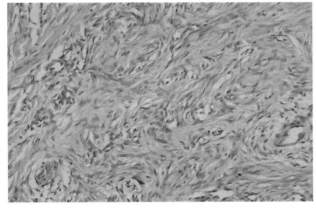

FIG. 25-30

Dermatofibrosarcoma protuberans. The fibroblasts are arranged in irregular intertwining bands. In some areas the cells radiate from a central hub of fibrous tissue in a whorllike fashion, resulting in a cartwheel pattern. (× 64)

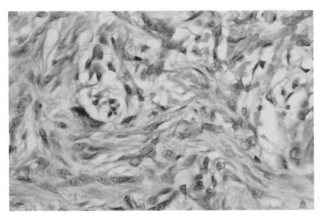

FIG. 25-31

Dermatofibrosarcoma protuberans. The nuclei of the fibroblasts lie in irregular strands and whorls. Some of the nuclei show a slight degree of atypicality. Formation of collagen is well in evidence. (× 160)

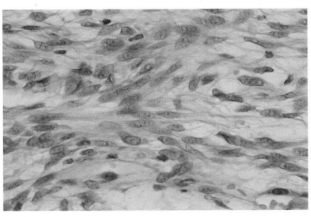

FIG. 25-32

Dermatofibrosarcoma protuberans. The cells have large, spindle-shaped nuclei and are arranged in bands. The nuclei show a moderate degree of atypicality. (× 160)

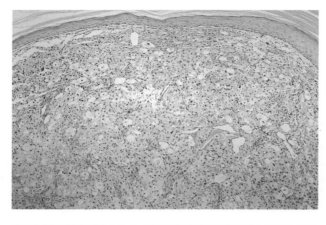

FIG. 25-33

Atypical fibroxanthoma. A highly cellular infiltrate extends close to the epidermis. The cells have a clear cytoplasm. (× 16)

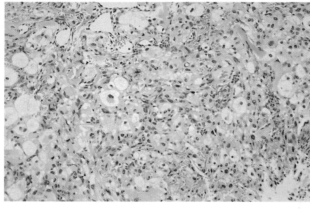

FIG. 25-34

Atypical fibroxanthoma. The infiltrate is composed of cells with pleomorphic nuclei and ample cytoplasm containing lipids. (× 40)

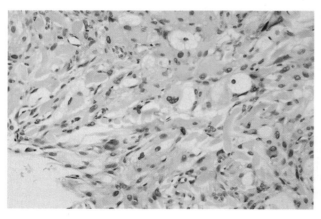

FIG. 25-35

Atypical fibroxanthoma. The cells appear polygonal and have ample, foamy, and vacuolated cytoplasm. Multinucleated giant cells are present. (× 64)

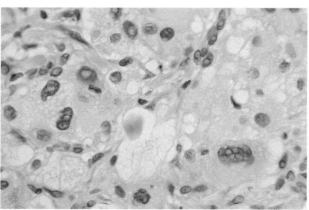

FIG. 25-36

Atypical fibroxanthoma. The atypical cells with hyperchromatic nuclei have a foamy cytoplasm. Many giant cells are present. (× 160)

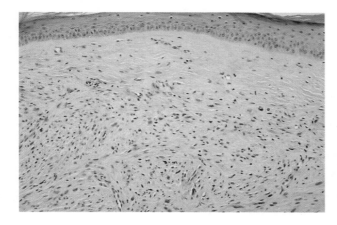

FIG. 25-37

Atypical fibroxanthoma. A highly cellular infiltrate extends close to the epidermis. Several atypical hyperchromatic nuclei can be recognized at this low magnification. (× 40)

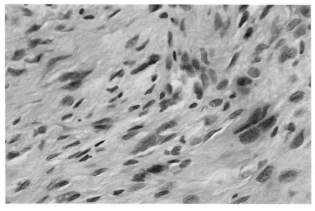

FIG. 25-38

Atypical fibroxanthoma. The atypical cells show pleomorphic, hyperchromatic nuclei. (× 160)

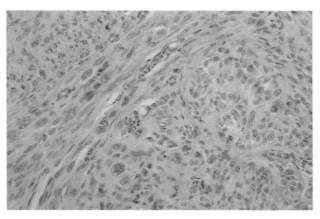

FIG. 25-39

Malignant fibrous histiocytoma. A highly cellular tumor with a pleomorphic appearance can be recognized. The atypical cells are arranged in an intertwining, storiform pattern. (× 64)

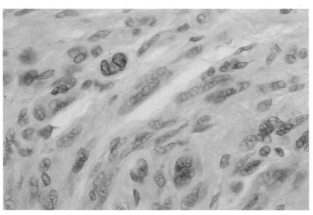

FIG. 25-40

Malignant fibrous histiocytoma. The cells show irregularly shaped nuclei. Multinucleated giant cells with bizarrely shaped, large, hyperchromatic nuclei are present. (× 160)

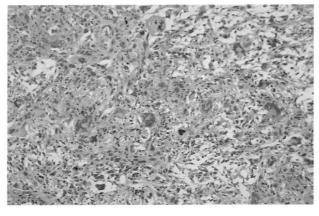

FIG. 25-41

Malignant fibrous histiocytoma (fibroxanthosarcoma). The pleomorphic dermal tumor shows several multinucleated giant cells. (× 40)

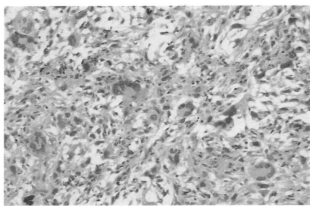

FIG. 25-42

Malignant fibrous histiocytoma (fibroxanthosarcoma), higher magnification of Fig. 25-41. Several bizarre giant cells are present. (× 64)

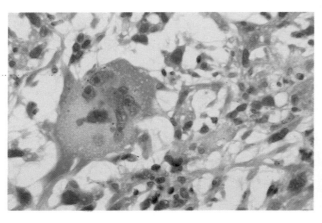

FIG. 25-43

Malignant fibrous histiocytoma (fibroxanthosarcoma). The giant cells show several nuclei with large nucleoli and ample cytoplasm that is vacuolated. (× 160)

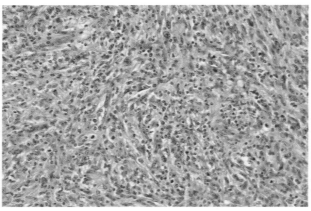

FIG. 25-44

Malignant fibrous histiocytoma. A highly cellular tumor with a pleomorphic appearance can be recognized. (× 64)

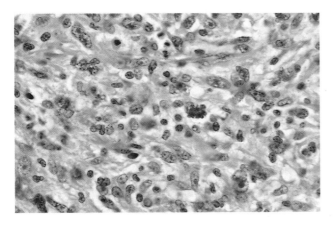

FIG. 25-45

Malignant fibrous histiocytoma. The atypical cells appear histiocytelike. An atypical mitosis can be recognized. (× 160)

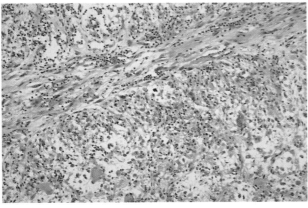

FIG. 25-46

Malignant fibrous histiocytoma, inflammatory variant. Atypical giant cells, in addition to an intense infiltrate of neutrophils, are present. (× 40)

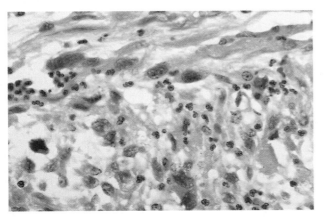

FIG. 25-47

Malignant fibrous histiocytoma, inflammatory variant. Numerous neutrophils can be recognized, in addition to atypical tumor cells. (× 160)

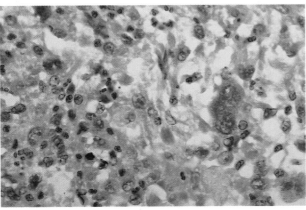

FIG. 25-48

Malignant fibrous histiocytoma, inflammatory variant. The tumor is composed of neutrophils, atypical histiocytes, and atypical giant cells. (× 160)

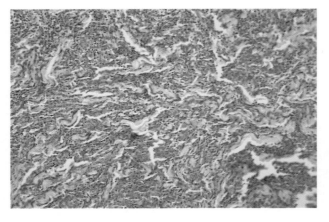

FIG. 25-49

Epithelioid sarcoma. The tumor consists of irregular nodular aggregates of tumor cells, embedded in fibrous tissue. (× 40)

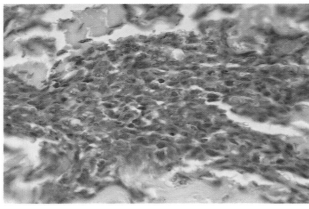

FIG. 25-50

Epithelioid sarcoma. The tumor cells lie in nodular aggregates. They have polygonal nuclei and abundant cytoplasm, thereby resembling epithelioid cells. Several of the nuclei are hyperchromatic. (× 160)

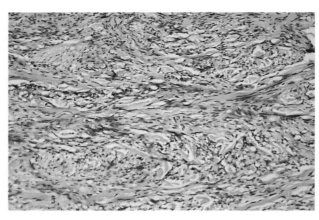

FIG. 25-51

Epithelioid sarcoma, incubation with monoclonal antibody against keratin. This tumor consists of spindle-shaped cells that contain keratin in their cytoplasm. APAAP technique. (× 40)

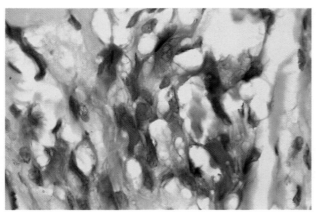

FIG. 25-52

Epithelioid sarcoma, higher magnification, incubation with monoclonal antibody against keratin. The tumor cells show a positive reaction. (× 240)

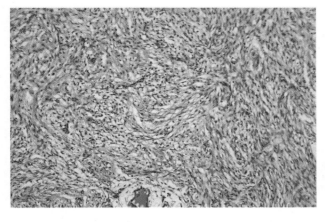

FIG. 25-53

Fibrosarcoma. The tumor consists of fascicles of atypical spindle cells. (× 16)

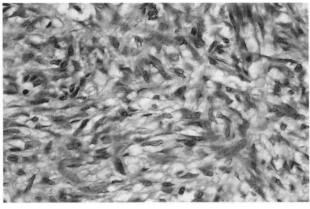

FIG. 25-54

Fibrosarcoma. The majority of tumor cells show spindle-shaped nuclei. (× 64)

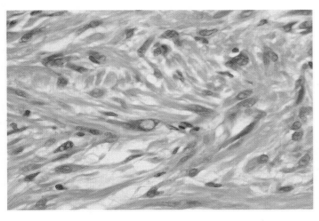

FIG. 25-55

Fibrosarcoma. Spindle-shaped tumor cells lie in parallel rows and are arranged in a herringbone pattern. (× 160)

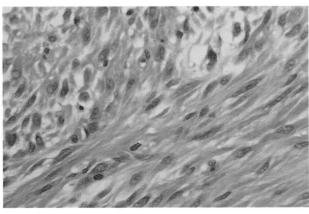

FIG. 25-56

Fibrosarcoma. The spindle-shaped tumor cells lie in parallel rows. (× 160)

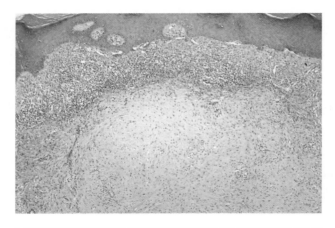

FIG. 25-57

Fibromyxoma. Within a localized area of the dermis the collagen is replaced by homogenous mucinous material. (× 16)

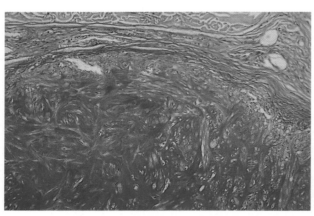

FIG. 25-58

Fibromyxoma, higher magnification. The number of mucoblasts is increased in early lesions mainly in the center, whereas, in older lesions (this photomicrograph), after mucin has accumulated, the increase in fibroblasts is largely evident at the base and on the sides of the lesion. (× 40)

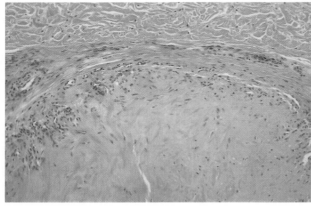

FIG. 25-59

Fibromyxoma, alcian stain. The mucinous material stains blue. (× 40)

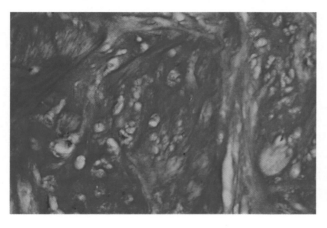

FIG. 25-60

Fibromyxoma, alcian stain, higher magnification. The mucinous material stains blue, whereas the nuclei of the mucoblasts stain red. Cleftlike spaces or small cavities are present within the mucinous material. (× 160)

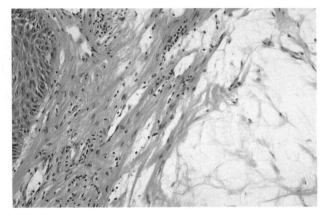

FIG. 25-61

Digital mucous cyst, early stage. Cleftlike spaces containing mucin are present. Through coalescence the cleftlike spaces will later form a large cystic space. (× 40)

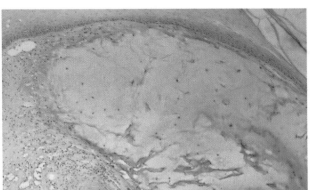

FIG. 25-62

Digital mucous cyst, alcian stain. The mucinous material present within the cyst stains blue. (× 16)

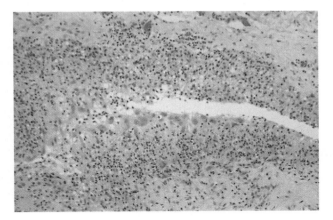

FIG. 25-63

Mucous cyst of the oral mucosa. The cyst is a result of the rupture of a salivary duct. The cavity contains sialomucin and is surrounded by granulation tissue. (× 40)

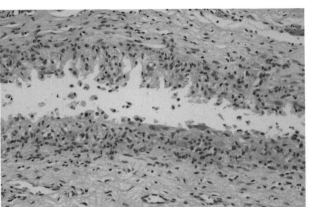

FIG. 25-64

Mucous cyst of the oral mucosa, higher magnification. The cystic space is lined by a thick layer of granulation tissue composed of lymphocytes, fibroblasts, macrophages, and capillaries. (× 64)

CHAPTER 26

Tumors of
Vascular Tissue

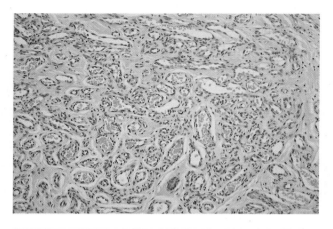

FIG. 26-1

Capillary hemangioma, mature lesion. The tumor consists of dilated capillaries with flattened endothelial cells. (× 16)

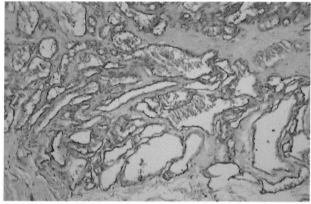

FIG. 26-2

Capillary hemangioma incubated with Ulex europaeus I, an endothelial marker. The endothelial cells show a positive reaction consisting of a dark brown line on the luminal surface (compare Fig. 2-15). (× 40)

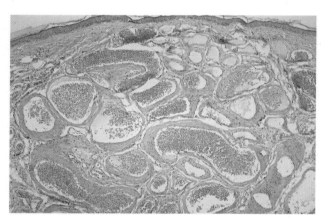

FIG. 26-3

Cavernous hemangioma. The tumor consists of large irregular lumina containing erythrocytes. The lumina are lined by a single layer of thin endothelial cells. The lumina are surrounded by a fibrous wall. (× 16)

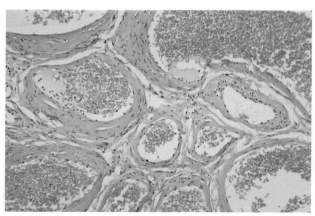

FIG. 26-4

Cavernous hemangioma, higher magnification. The dilated lumina are surrounded by a thick fibrous wall. (× 40)

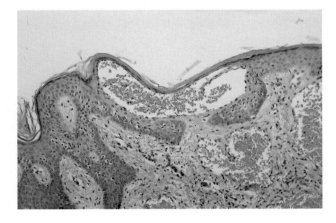

FIG. 26-5

Angiokeratoma circumscriptum. Greatly dilated capillary spaces are seen in the papillary and reticular dermis. The capillaries are filled with erythrocytes. (× 40)

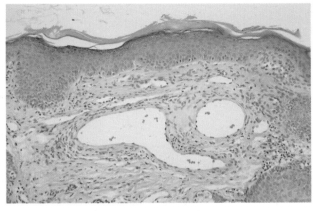

FIG. 26-6

Nevus araneus. The center of the lesion shows a single ascending artery, the wall of which shows smooth muscle. (× 40)

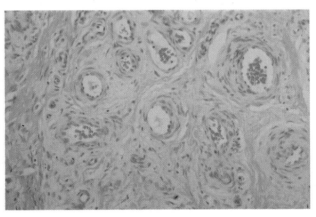

FIG. 26-7

Venous hemangioma. Within the dermis densely aggregated, thick-walled and thin-walled vessels lined by a single layer of endothelial cells can be seen. (× 64)

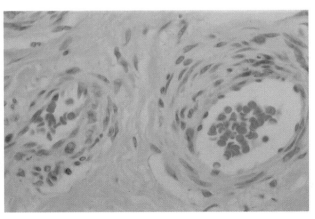

FIG. 26-8

Venous hemangioma, higher magnification. The walls of the thick-walled vessels mainly consist of fibrous tissue but in most instances also contain some smooth muscle. (× 160)

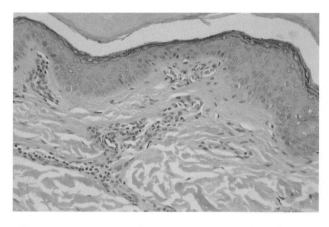

FIG. 26-9

Superficial essential telangiectasia. Dilated vessels are seen immediately beneath the epidermis. ($\times$ 64)

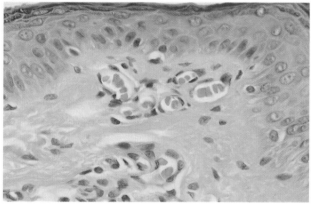

FIG. 26-10

Superficial essential telangiectasia, higher magnification. The walls of the vessels are composed only of endothelium. ($\times$ 160)

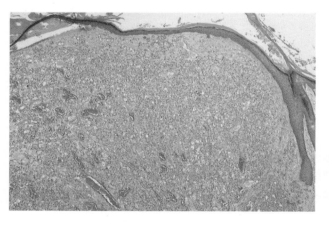

FIG. 26-11

Granuloma pyogenicum. The lesion that is covered by a flattened epidermis consists of endothelial proliferations with formation of capillary lumina. On the right, part of the epidermal collarette is seen. ($\times$ 10)

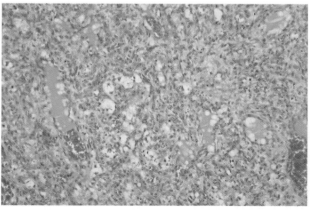

FIG. 26-12

Granuloma pyogenicum. The lesion consists of endothelial proliferations with capillary lumina. ($\times$ 40)

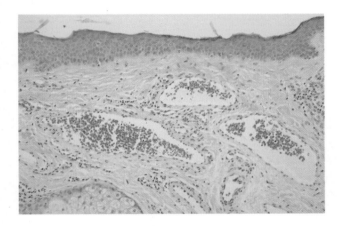

FIG. 26-13

Venous lake. The lesion consists of dilated veins or venules. They are lined by a single layer of flattened endothelial cells and a thin wall of fibrous tissue. (× 40)

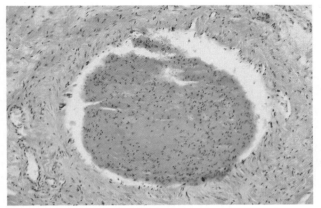

FIG. 26-14

Thrombosed vein. A greatly dilated vascular lumen is filled with a thrombus that has been invaded by fibroblasts, indicating beginning organization. (× 40)

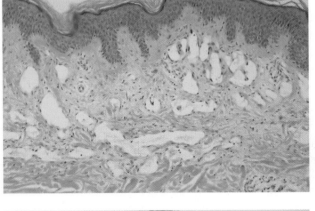

FIG. 26-15

Lymphangioma circumscriptum. Greatly dilated lymph vessels lined by a single layer of endothelium are present in the uppermost portion of the dermis. (× 40)

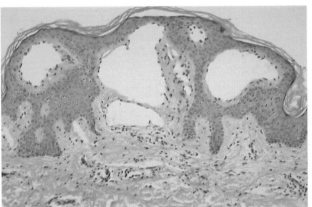

FIG. 26-16

Lymphangioma circumscriptum. Dilated lymph vessels lined by a single layer of endothelium are present in the upper portion of the dermis. The epidermis shows downward growth and surrounds some of the lymph vessels. (× 40)

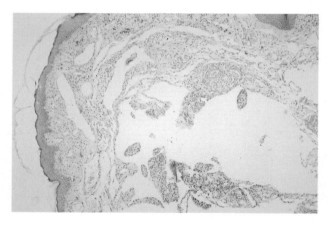

FIG. 26-17

Cavernous lymphangioma. Large, irregularly shaped cystic spaces are seen throughout the dermis. They are lined by a single layer of endothelial cells. (× 16)

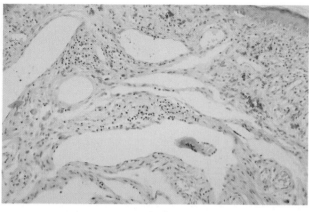

FIG. 26-18

Cavernous lymphangioma. The large cystic spaces are surrounded by loose stroma. (× 40)

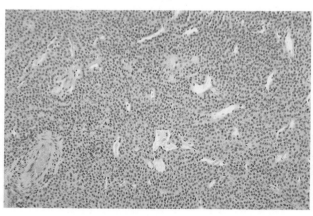

FIG. 26-19

Solitary glomus tumor. These tumors contain numerous small vascular lumina lined by a single layer of flattened endothelial cells. Peripheral to the endothelial cells are many layers of glomus cells. (× 40)

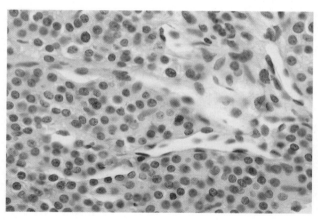

FIG. 26-20

Solitary glomus tumor, higher magnification. The lumina contain flattened endothelial cells and are surrounded by multiple layers of glomus cells. The glomus cells have round to oval nuclei of a rather uniform appearance. They resemble epithelioid cells. (× 160)

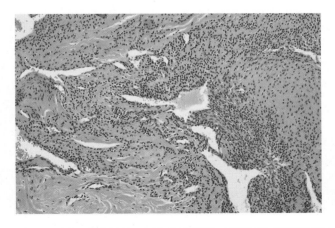

FIG. 26-21

Solitary glomus tumor. Several dilated lumina are present that are surrounded by multiple layers of glomus cells. (× 40)

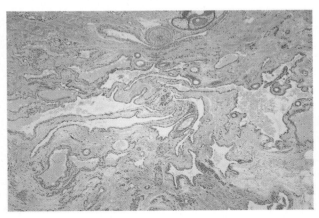

FIG. 26-22

Solitary glomus tumor. The glomus cells have a faintly eosinophilic cytoplasm and large, round to oval nuclei of a rather uniform appearance. The stroma appears edematous. (× 160)

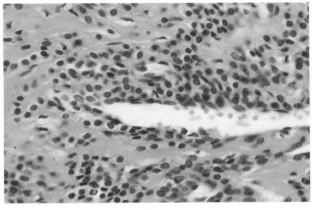

FIG. 26-23

Multiple glomus tumor. The vascular spaces are larger than in the solitary lesion. The large vascular spaces are lined by flattened endothelium. Peripheral to the endothelial cells a narrow rim of one to three layers of glomus cells is seen. (× 16)

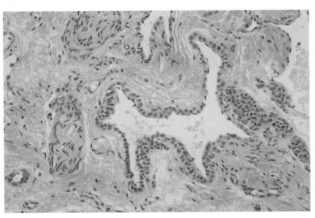

FIG. 26-24

Multiple glomus tumor. The central large vascular space has an irregular shape, is lined by a single layer of flattened endothelial cells, and is surrounded by one to three layers of glomus cells. (× 64)

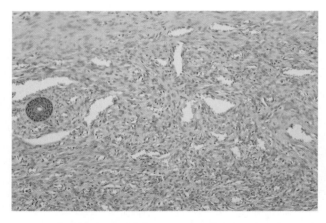

FIG. 26-25

Hemangiopericytoma. The tumor consists of endothelium-lined tubes and sprouts surrounded by irregularly proliferating, closely packed pericytes. (Courtesy of W. Nikolowski, M.D.) (× 40)

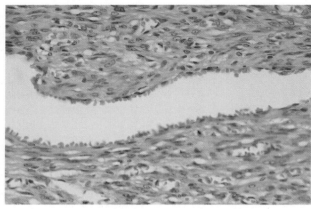

FIG. 26-26

Hemangiopericytoma. The vascular lumen is lined by flattened endothelial cells that are surrounded by irregularly proliferating, closely packed pericytes with spindle-shaped nuclei. (Courtesy of W. Nikolowski, M.D.) (× 100)

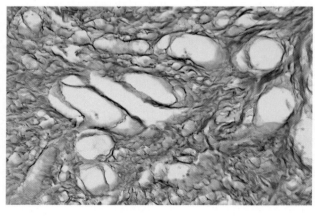

FIG. 26-27

Hemangiopericytoma, reticulum stain. The reticulum fibers encircle the capillary endothelium. The tumor cells are seen to be located peripheral to the periendothelial ring of reticulum. The section was counterstained with methylene green. (× 100)

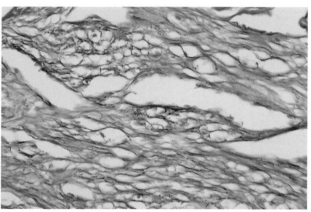

FIG. 26-28

Hemangioperictyoma, reticulum stain. The individual tumor cells are surrounded by a delicate network of reticulum fibers. (× 100)

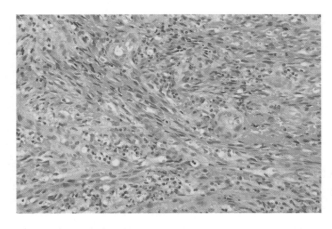

FIG. 26-29

Kaposi's sarcoma. The tumor consists of spindle cell formations containing vascular slits. (× 64)

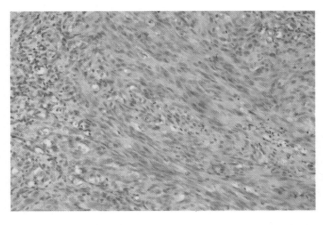

FIG. 26-30

Kaposi's sarcoma. Strands of atypical spindle cells are seen containing vascular formations and small groups of extravasated erythrocytes. (× 160)

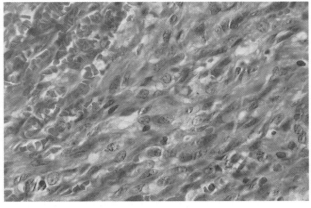

FIG. 26-31

Kaposi's sarcoma, incubation with Ulex europaeus I, an endothelial marker. About half of the tumor cells show a positive reaction within the cytoplasm. PAP technique. (× 64)

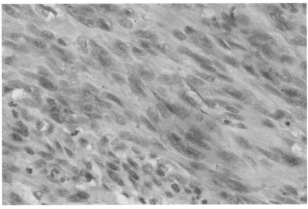

FIG. 26-32

Kaposi's sarcoma, higher magnification of Fig. 26-31. Incubation with the endothelial marker Ulex europaeus I shows a positive reaction within the cytoplasm of the atypical cells. PAP technique. (× 160)

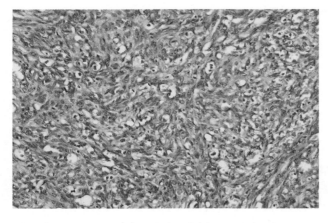

FIG. 26-33

Kaposi's sarcoma. A diffuse infiltration of endothelial cells with extravasated erythrocytes is seen. (× 64)

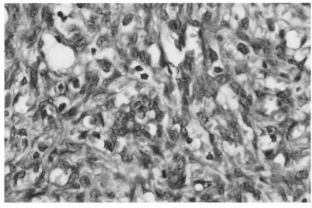

FIG. 26-34

Kaposi's sarcoma, higher magnification of Fig. 26-33. The tumor consists of endothelial cells and extravasated erythrocytes. (× 160)

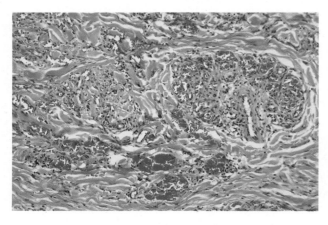

FIG. 26-35

Kaposi's sarcoma, early lesion from a patient with the acquired immunodeficiency syndrome (AIDS). The lesion consists of widely dilated, thin-walled capillaries. The lesion thus resembles granulation tissue. (× 40)

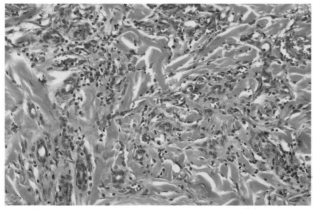

FIG. 26-36

Kaposi's sarcoma, early lesion, higher magnification of Fig. 26-35. The capillaries are dilated and increased in number. A diffuse chronic inflammatory infiltrate is present. (× 64)

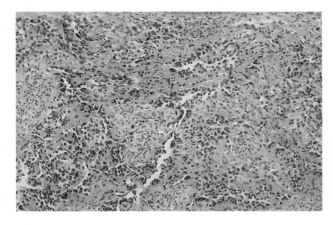

FIG. 26-37

Angiosarcoma of the elderly. The tumor shows vascular spaces lined by atypical, cuboidal endothelial cells. Between the vascular spaces, solid proliferations of more or less cuboidal endothelial cells are seen. (× 40)

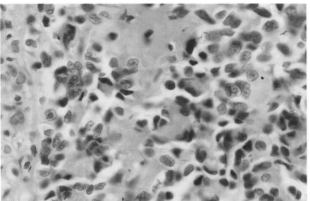

FIG. 26-38

Angiosarcoma of the elderly. The tumor cells are frankly atypical, cuboidal endothelial cells. (× 160)

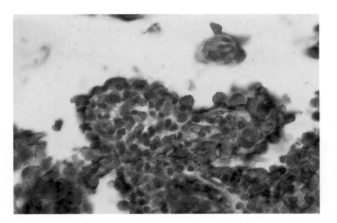

FIG. 26-39

Angiosarcoma of the elderly, incubation with the endothelial marker Ulex europaeus I. A vascular channel is lined by several layers of endothelial cells (right side of the photomicrograph). The positive reaction product of Ulex is orange-brown and is located in the plasma membrane. PAP technique. (× 160)

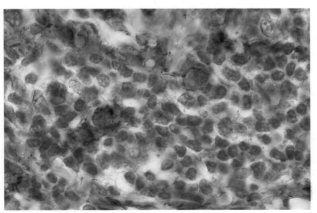

FIG. 26-40

Angiosarcoma of the elderly, incubation with the endothelial marker Ulex europaeus I. Within a solid area of tumor cells a few cells show a positive reaction with Ulex. (× 240)

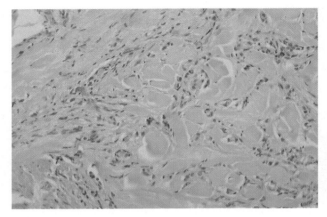

FIG. 26-41

Angiosarcoma secondary to persistent chronic lymphedema (Stewart-Treves syndrome). Narrow strands of proliferating, atypical endothelial cells are present. (× 40)

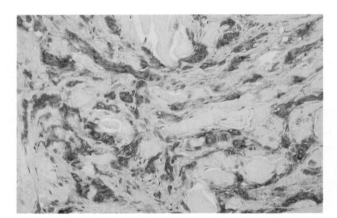

FIG. 26-42

Angiosarcoma secondary to persistent chronic lymphedema (Stewart-Treves syndrome). Narrow strands of atypical endothelial cells are present. No vascular lumina can be recognized. (× 40)

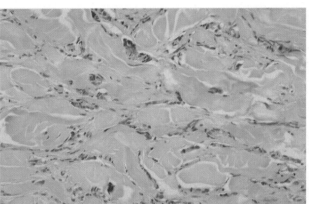

FIG. 26-43

Angiosarcoma secondary to persistent chronic lymphedema (Stewart-Treves syndrome). Incubation with the endothelial marker Ulex europaeus I helps to identify the tumor cells as endothelial cells. PAP technique. (× 64)

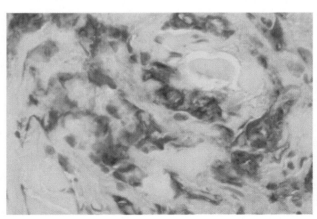

FIG. 26-44

Angiosarcoma secondary to persistent chronic lymphedema (Stewart-Treves syndrome). The tumor cells show a positive reaction when incubated with Ulex europaeus. PAP technique. (× 160)

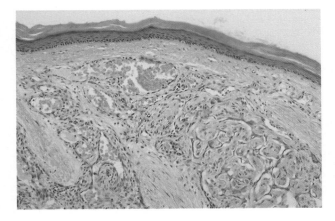

FIG. 26-45

Malignant proliferating angioendotheliomatosis (intravascular B cell lymphoma). The capillaries are dilated and partially filled with proliferated cells that look like endothelial cells, but are B lymphoma cells. (× 40)

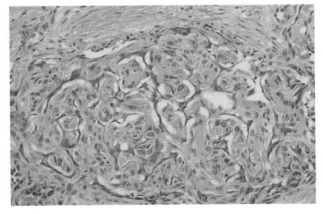

FIG. 26-46

Malignant proliferating angioendotheliomatosis (intravascular B cell lymphoma). The capillaries are filled with atypical cells that are B lymphoma cells. (× 64)

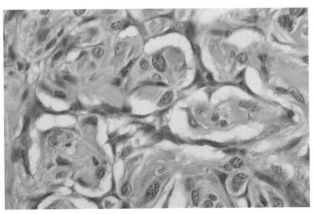

FIG. 26-47

Malignant proliferating angioendotheliomatosis (intravascular B cell lymphoma). The lumina are almost occluded with atypical B cells. (× 160)

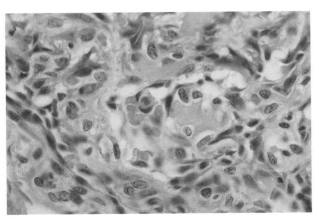

FIG. 26-48

Malignant proliferating angioendotheliomatosis (intravascular B cell lymphoma). A few erythrocytes can be seen in the vascular lumina that are otherwise occluded with atypical B cells. (× 160)

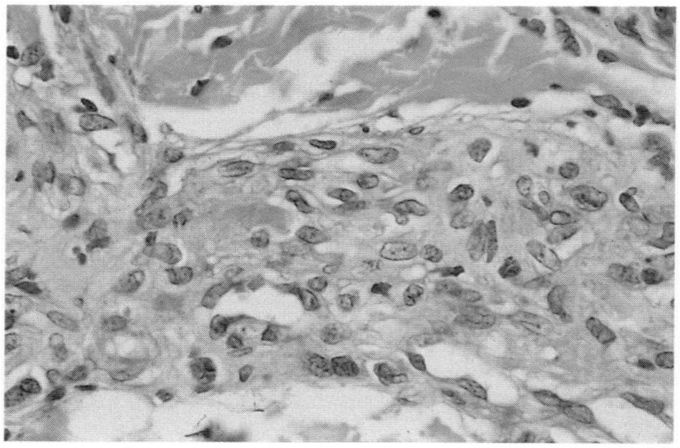

FIG. 26-49

Reactive proliferating angioendotheliomatosis. The capillaries are completely filled with proliferating endothelial cells showing no atypicality. (× 160)

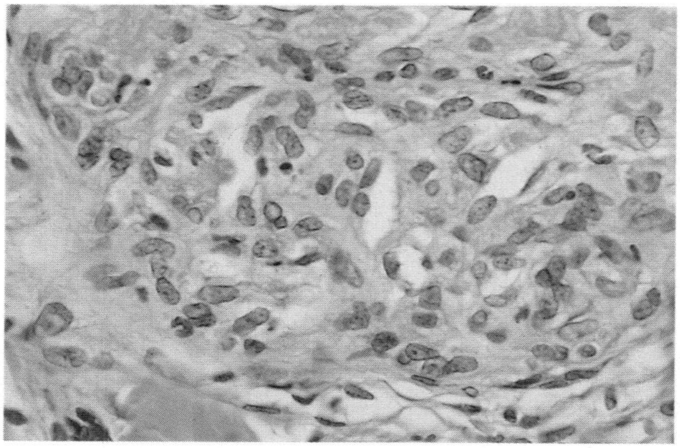

FIG. 26-50

Reactive proliferating angioendotheliomatosis. The capillaries are dilated and show considerable proliferation of benign endothelial cells. (× 160)

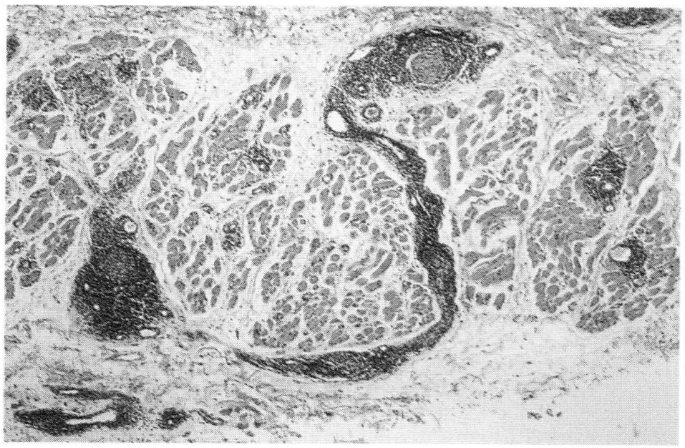

FIG. 26-51

Angiolymphoid hyperplasia. The capillaries are lined by swollen, endothelial cells that protrude into the lumen and are surrounded by lymphocytes. (× 16)

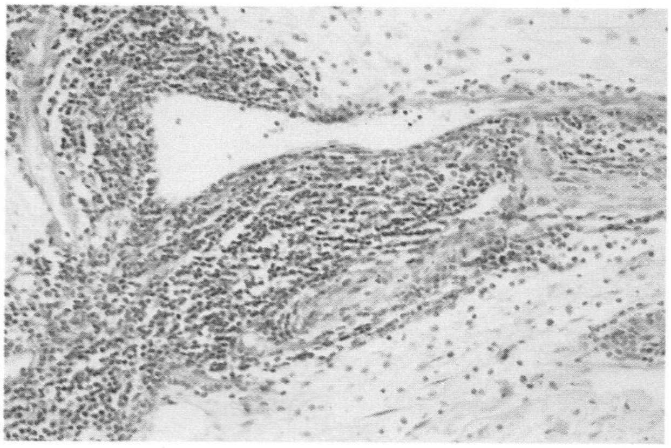

FIG. 26-52

Angiolymphoid hyperplasia, Giemsa stain. There is an extensive perivascular infiltrate of lymphocytes and histiocytes. Eosinophils usually are prominent in the infiltrate, but they may be few in number or can even be absent. (× 160)

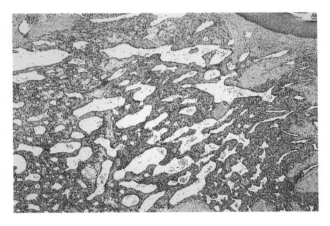

FIG. 26-53

Intravascular papillary endothelial hyperplasia (Masson's pseudoangiosarcoma). Irregular connective tissue stalks are lined with a single layer of endothelial cells. (× 16)

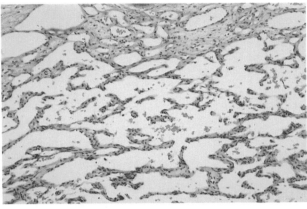

FIG. 26-54

Intravascular papillary endothelial hyperplasia (Masson's pseudoangiosarcoma). Within a vascular lumen a network of connective tissue stalks can be seen that is lined by endothelium. (× 40)

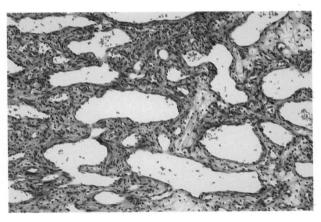

FIG. 26-55

Intravascular papillary endothelial hyperplasia (Masson's pseudoangiosarcoma). The irregular connective tissue stalks are lined with one layer of endothelial cells. Erythrocytes are seen within the irregular luminal spaces. (× 40)

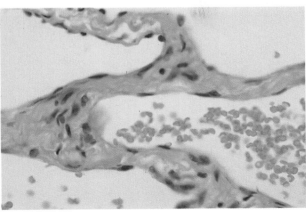

FIG. 26-56

Intravascular papillary endothelial hyperplasia (Masson's pseudoangiosarcoma), higher magnification of a connective tissue stalk showing the endothelial lining. (× 160)

CHAPTER 27

Tumors of Fatty, Muscular, and Osseous Tissue

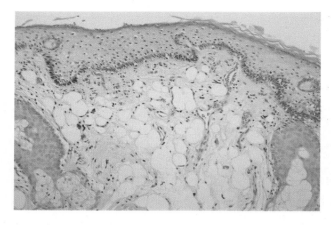

FIG. 27-1

Nevus lipomatosus superficialis. Groups and strands of fat cells are found embedded among the collagen bundles of the dermis, as high as the papillary dermis. (× 40)

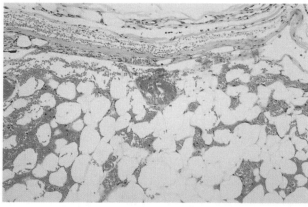

FIG. 27-2

Angiolipoma. The lesion consists of mature adipose tissue and a varying number of blood vessels. (× 40)

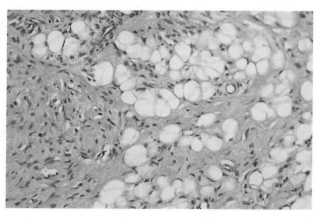

FIG. 27-3

Fibrolipoma. The lesion consists of mature fat cells and mature collagen containing many fibroblasts. The collagen has invaded the fatty tissue. (× 64)

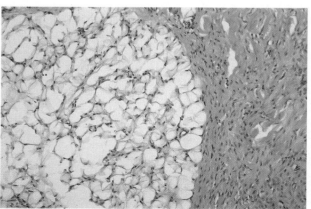

FIG. 27-4

Fibrolipoma. On the right-hand side mature collagen containing many fibroblasts can be seen. On the left-hand side mature adipose tissue with collagen surrounding each fat cell is visible. (× 40)

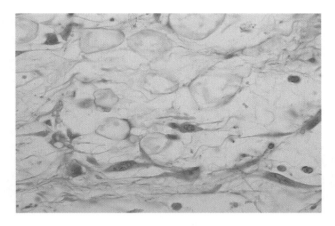

FIG. 27·5

Liposarcoma. The tumor is composed of lipoblasts showing spindle-shaped nuclei, but it also contains mature fat cells. (× 160)

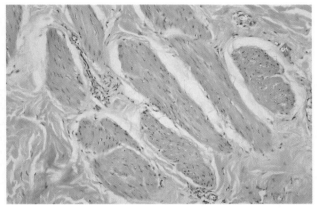

FIG. 27·6

Piloleiomyoma. The tumor consists of several bundles of smooth muscle fibers. Collagen bundles can be seen between muscle bundles. Both stain alike with hemotoxylin. (× 40)

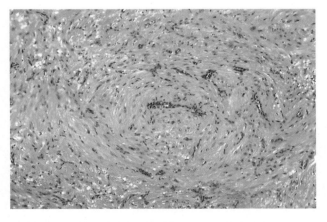

FIG. 27·7

Angioleiomyoma. A large vein is present with only a slitlike lumen. Smooth muscle bundles extend tangentially from the periphery of the vein and merge with intervascular muscle bundles. (× 40)

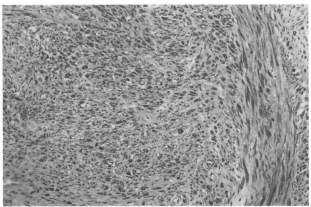

FIG. 27·8

Angioleiomyoma, Masson's trichrome stain. The muscles and their nuclei stain red, the collagen blue. (× 64)

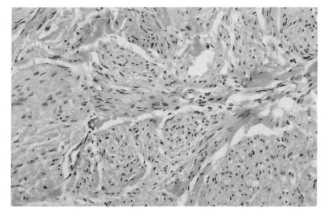

FIG. 27-9

Leiomyosarcoma. The tumor shows nodular aggregates and densely packed, interlacing bundles of smooth muscle cells. (× 64)

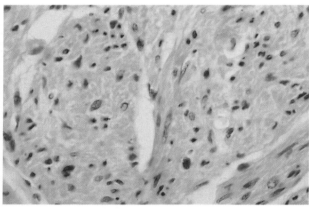

FIG. 27-10

Leiomyosarcoma. Several large, plump nuclei can be seen within rather well-demarcated muscle bundles. The nuclei are located within the center of the muscle cell. (× 160)

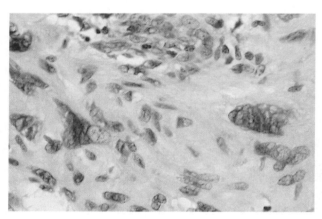

FIG. 27-11

Leiomyosarcoma, higher magnification. Several irregularly shaped, anaplastic nuclei and atypical giant cells with bizarre nuclei can be seen. (× 160)

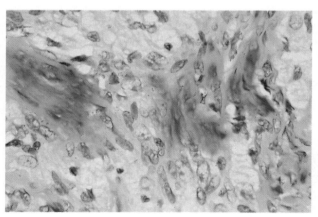

FIG. 27-12

Leiomyosarcoma, incubated with anti-desmin, one of the cytoskeletal filaments present in muscle cells. The tumor cells show a positive reaction. (× 160)

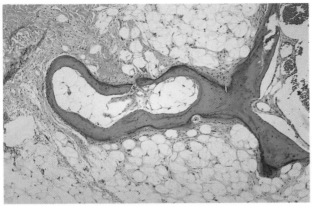

FIG. 27·13

Osteoma cutis. Within the subcutaneous fat, bone is present. The bone contains cement lines. ($\times$ 16)

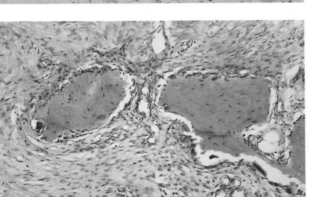

FIG. 27·14

Osteoma cutis. Osteoblasts with elongated nuclei are present at the periphery of the bone where new bone is being laid down. Osteoclasts are present in the left piece of bone. They lie within a niche called Howship's lacuna. ($\times$ 40)

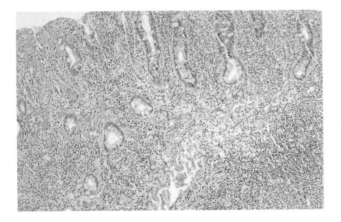

FIG. 27·15

Umbilical omphalomesenteric duct polyp. Ectopic gastrointestinal epithelium is present on the surface of the umbilical polyp. It represents remnants of the omphalomesenteric duct. The gastrointestinal epithelium in this polyp has the appearance of the colonic mucosa. ($\times$ 16)

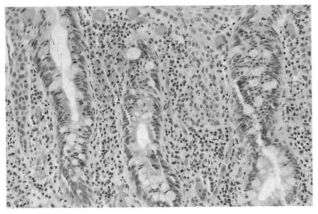

FIG. 27·16

Umbilical omphalomesenteric duct polyp, higher magnification. The gastrointestinal polyp has the appearance of colonic mucosa. The polyp also shows proliferated capillaries and a diffuse chronic inflammatory infiltrate. ($\times$ 40)

C H A P T E R 28

Tumors of
Neural Tissue

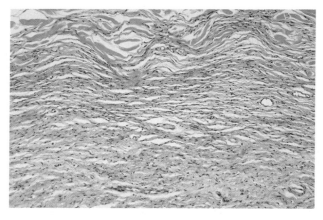

FIG. 28-1

Neurofibroma. The lesion consists of faintly eosinophilic, thin, wavy fibers lying in loosely textured strands. Within the fibers a fairly large number of long spindle-shaped nuclei can be seen. (× 40)

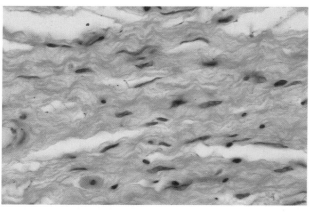

FIG. 28-2

Neurofibroma, higher magnification of Fig. 28-1. The lesion is composed of long, wavy fibers with elongated nuclei. (× 240)

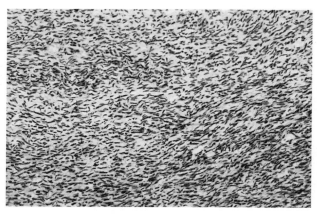

FIG. 28-3

Neurofibrosarcoma. The number of nuclei is increased and the nuclei are atypical. The wavy pattern is preserved. (× 64)

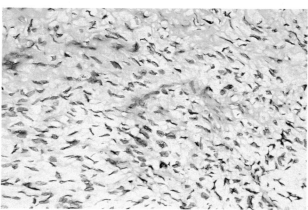

FIG. 28-4

Neurofibrosarcoma. Incubation with a monoclonal antibody against neurofilaments shows a positive reaction in some of the tumor cells. APAAP technique. (× 160)

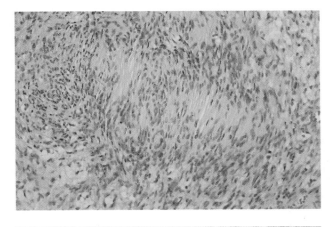

FIG. 28-5

Neurilemmoma. The tumor is composed of cells with elongated and tightly packed nuclei. ($\times$ 64)

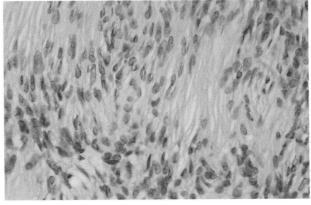

FIG. 28-6

Neurilemmoma. The tumor consists of Schwann cells that have elongated nuclei and long processes. ($\times$ 160)

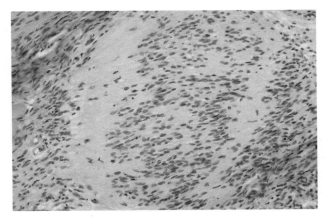

FIG. 28-7

Neurilemmoma. A highly characteristic feature is the arrangement of the nuclei in two parallel rows, enclosing between them a space of nearly homogenous anucleate material. These formations are called Verocay bodies. ($\times$ 64)

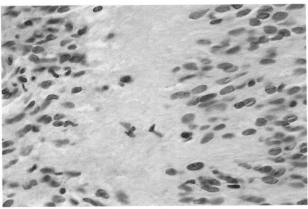

FIG. 28-8

Neurilemmoma, higher magnification. A Verocay body is shown, consisting of two rows of nuclei with a space of homogeneous anucleate material between them. ($\times$ 160)

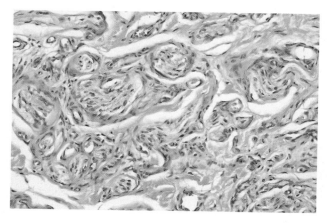

FIG. 28-9

Neuroma from a rudimentary supernumerary digit. Large bundles of nerves are present. They are surrounded by a capsule formed by perineurial cells and collagen. (× 64)

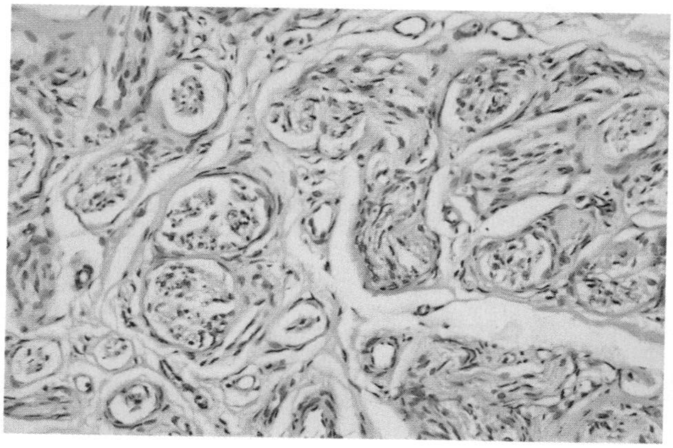

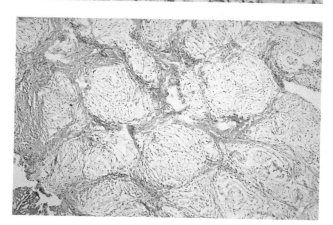

FIG. 28-10

Neuroma incubated with a monoclonal antibody against neurofilaments. The nerves give a positive reaction by staining red. APAAP technique. (× 64)

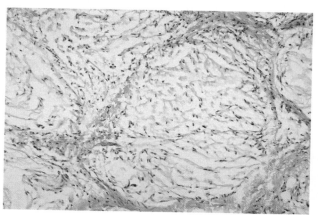

FIG. 28-11

Pacinian neurofibroma. The tumor contains numerous round or ovoid lobules, each showing a central homogenous eosionphilic core surrounded by as many as 30 pale-staining concentric collagenous lamellae. (× 16)

FIG. 28-12

Pacinian neurofibroma. The lobules contain numerous elliptic or spindle-shaped nuclei both in the central core and in the surrounding lamellae. (× 40)

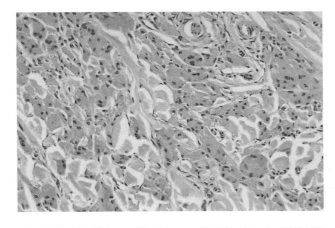

FIG. 28-13

Granular cell tumor. The large tumor cells are filled with coarse granules. ($\times$ 64)

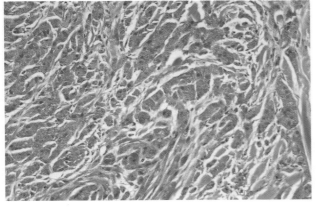

FIG. 28-14

Granular cell tumor, PAS stain. The cytoplasmic granules are PAS positive and diastase resistant. ($\times$ 64)

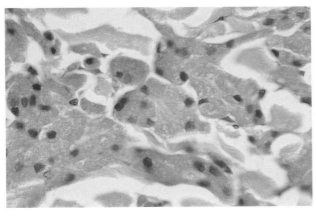

FIG. 28-15

Granular cell tumor. The tumor is composed of large cells with a pale cytoplasm filled with numerous fine granules. ($\times$ 160)

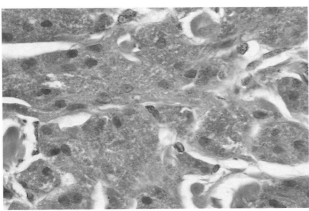

FIG. 28-16

Granular cell tumor, PAS stain. The tumor cells contain PAS-positive granules. ($\times$ 160)

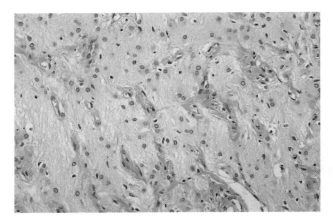

FIG. 28-17

Nasal glioma. The lesion shows loosely textured glial tissue with two types of cells: glial cells or astrocytes and neurons. ($\times$ 64)

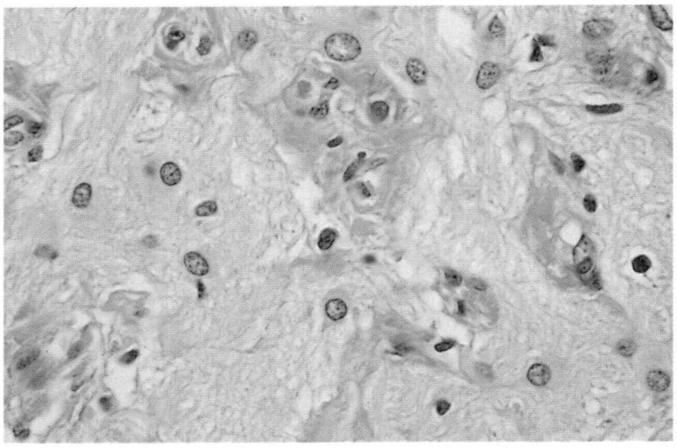

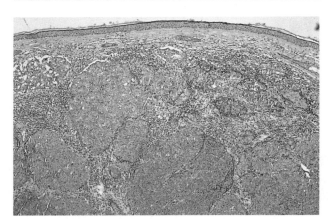

FIG. 28-18

Nasal glioma. The neurons show an eccentric nucleus and ample cytoplasm. The astrocytes possess oval nuclei. ($\times$ 160)

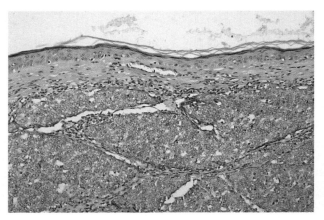

FIG. 28-19

Merkel cell carcinoma. The tumor consists of clusters of tumor cells in the dermis extending into the subcutis. ($\times$ 16)

FIG. 28-20

Merkel cell carcinoma. The tumor cells have a uniform appearance with closely spaced, round, vesicular nuclei and scanty ill-defined cytoplasm. ($\times$ 40)

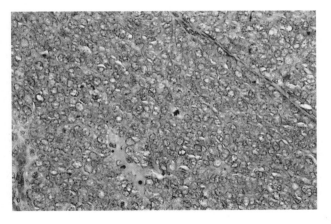

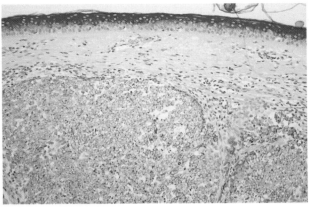

FIG. 28-21

Merkel cell carcinoma. Numerous mitotic figures are present showing a small, dark center surrounded by a clear space. (× 100)

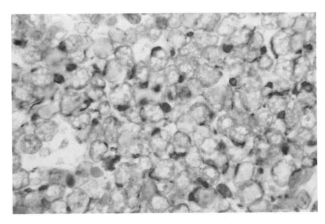

FIG. 28-22

Merkel cell carcinoma, incubation with a monoclonal antibody against keratin. The overlying epidermis shows uniform labeling, whereas the tumor cells contain keratin as fine globules. APAAP technique. (× 40)

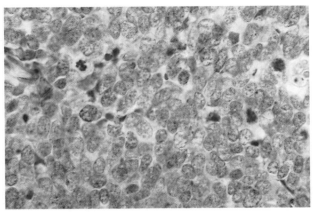

FIG. 28-23

Merkel cell carcinoma, incubation with a monoclonal antibody against keratin. Keratin is present as globular structures within the tumor cells. APAAP technique. (× 240)

FIG. 28-24

Merkel cell carcinoma, incubation with a monoclonal antibody against neurofilaments. Several tumor cells show a positive reaction consisting of globules in the cytoplasm. ABC technique. (× 240)

C H A P T E R   29

Melanocytic
Nevi and
Malignant
Melanoma

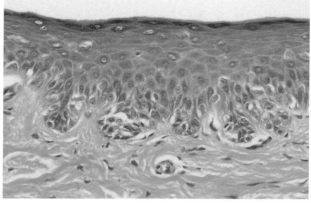

FIG. 29-1

Junction nevus. At the dermal–epidermal junction nevus cells lie in well-circumscribed nests. (× 64)

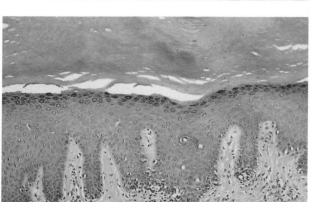

FIG. 29-2

Junction nevus from the sole of the foot. Well-circumscribed nests of nevus cells are seen in the tips of the rete ridges. (× 40)

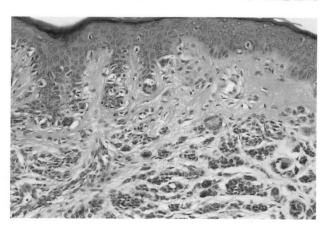

FIG. 29-3

Compound nevus. Nevus cell nests are seen at the dermal-epidermal junction and in the upper dermis. The nevus cells in the middermis are smaller than within the epidermis, and they contain less melanin than the junctional nevus cell nests. (× 40)

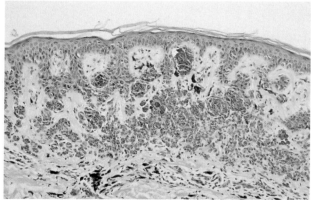

FIG. 29-4

Compound nevus. Nevus cell nests are present at the dermal-epidermal junction and in the upper dermis. The dermal nevus cells are cuboidal and distinctly smaller than the junctional nevus cells. This decrease in size and the good nesting are considered as maturation and are regarded as evidence of benignity. (× 64)

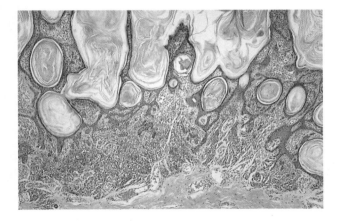

FIG. 29-5

Papillomatous compound nevus. The epidermis shows hyperkeratosis and papillomatosis as well as lacelike downward growth of epidermal strands and horn cysts. Nevus cell nests are present at the dermal-epidermal junction and in the dermis. ($\times$ 16)

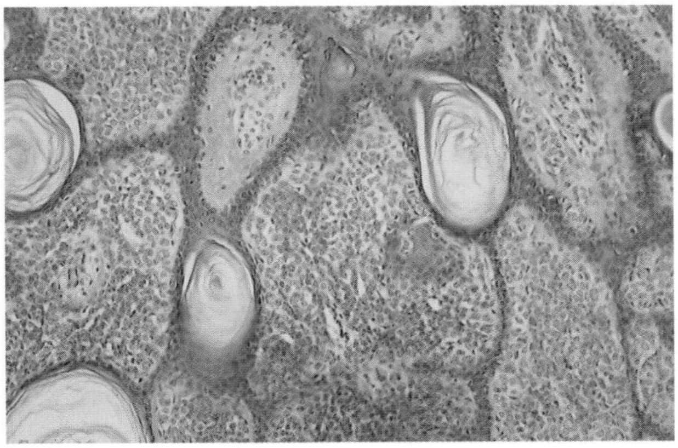

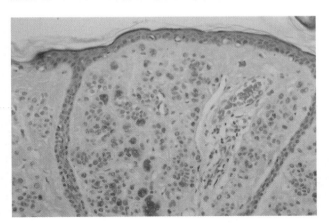

FIG. 29-6

Papillomatous compound nevus. The epidermis shows a lacelike downward growth and contains horn cysts. Nevus cell nests are found at the dermal-epidermal junction and in the corium. ($\times$ 40)

FIG. 29-7

Intradermal nevus. The upper dermis shows nests of nevus cells. Within the nests multinucleated nevus cells are seen in which small nuclei lie either in a rosettelike arrangement or close together in the center of the cell. These giant cells occur only in well matured nevi. ($\times$ 64)

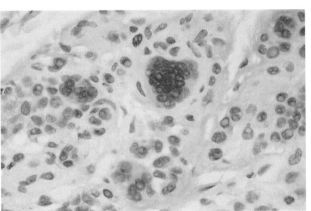

FIG. 29-8

Intradermal nevus with several multinucleated giant cells. The nuclei lie close together in the center of the cell. ($\times$ 160)

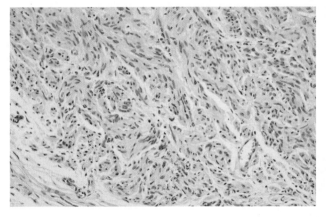

FIG. 29·9

Neural nevus. Spindle-shaped nevus cells are embedded in loosely arranged collagenous tissue. (× 64)

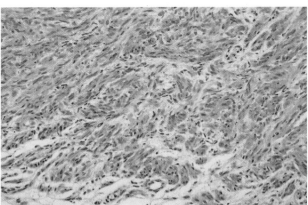

FIG. 29·10

Neural nevus, incubation with antibody against S 100 protein. The nevus cells show a positive reaction, as do all types of nevus cells. PAP technique. (× 64)

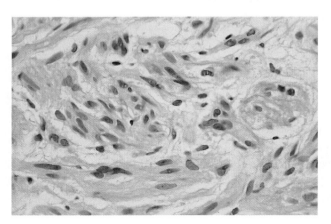

FIG. 29·11

Neural nevus. Spindle-shaped nevus cells are embedded in abundant, loosely arranged collagenous tissue. (× 160)

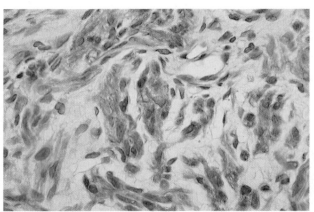

FIG. 29·12

Neural nevus. Incubation with antibody against S 100 protein shows a positive reaction. PAP technique. (× 160)

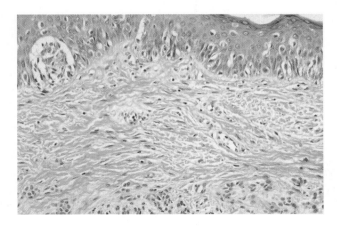

FIG. 29-13

Pseudomelanoma. Intraepidermal proliferation and hyperplasia of melanocytes is seen within the epidermis. This is a recurrent lesion with remnants of nevus cells in the lower part of the picture. (× 40)

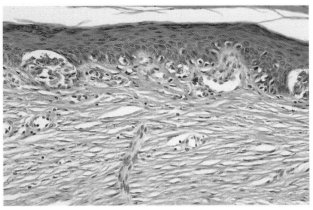

FIG. 29-14

Pseudomelanoma. Nevus cells, both singly and in nests are seen along the dermal-epidermal junction. Several nuclei are hyperchromatic. The dermis shows concentric layers of collagen. (× 40)

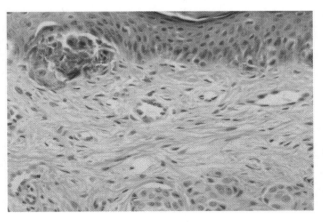

FIG. 29-15

Pseudomelanoma. At the dermal-epidermal junction nevus cell nests with hyperchromatic nuclei are present. Directly beneath the epidermis scar tissue is present, and immediately underneath the incompletely removed nevus is apparent. (× 64)

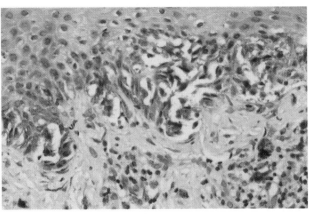

FIG. 29-16

Pseudomelanoma. At the dermal-epidermal junction a considerable number of nevus cells, both singly and in nests, are seen. A chronic inflammatory infiltrate containing melanophages is present in the upper dermis. (× 64)

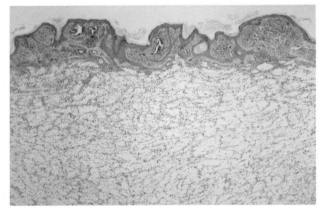

FIG. 29-17

Balloon cell nevus. Ballooned melanocytes are present in the upper dermis. (× 16)

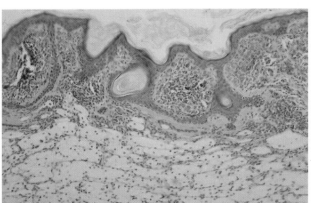

FIG. 29-18

Balloon cell nevus, higher magnification of Fig. 29-17. At the dermal-epidermal junction nests of nonballooned, moderately pigmented melanocytes are present. In the upper dermis ballooned melanocytes are aggregated. (× 40)

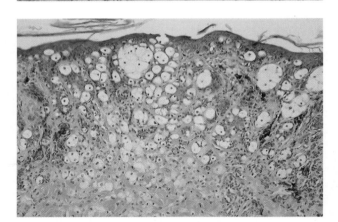

FIG. 29-19

Balloon cell nevus. At the dermal-epidermal junction and in the upper dermis nevus cell nests are present that mainly consist of ballooned melanocytes. (× 40)

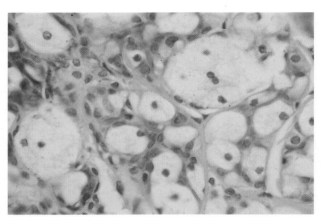

FIG. 29-20

Balloon cell nevus, higher magnification of Fig. 29-19. Balloon cells are considerably larger than ordinary nevus cells. Their nucleus is small, round, and usually centrally placed. (× 160)

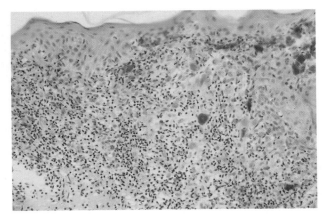

FIG. 29-21

Halo nevus. A dense lymphocytic infiltrate is present in the upper dermis and has partially invaded the epidermis. Between the lymphocytic cells scattered melanocytes can be recognized. (× 64)

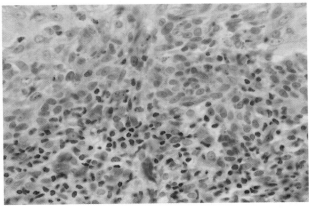

FIG. 29-22

Halo nevus, higher magnification of Fig. 29-21. Melanocytes and melanophages are scattered between lymphocytic cells. The melanophages are larger than the melanocytes and their melanin granules are coarser. (× 160)

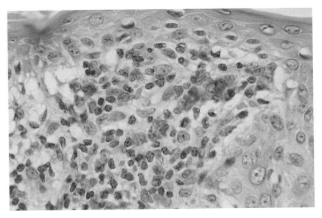

FIG. 29-23

Halo nevus. A nevus cell nest at the dermal-epidermal junction has been invaded by lymphocytes. Only a few melanocytes are still present. (× 160)

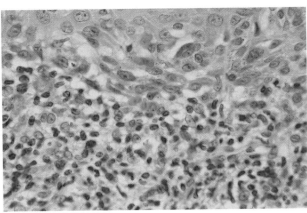

FIG. 29-24

Halo nevus. In the upper part of the photomicrograph a few slightly pigmented melanocytes are present, but the majority of cells are lymphocytes. (× 160)

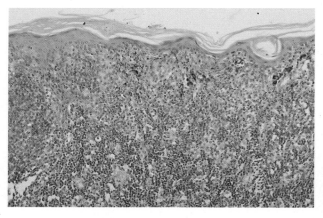

FIG. 29-25

Halo nevus. The dermis shows a dense lymphocytic infiltrate with a few scattered melanocytes present. ($\times$ 40)

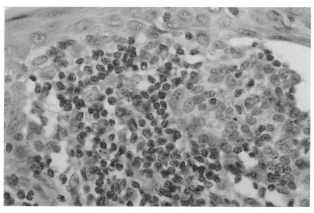

FIG. 29-26

Halo nevus, higher magnification. One junctional nevus cell nest is still present but being attacked by lymphocytes. ($\times$ 160)

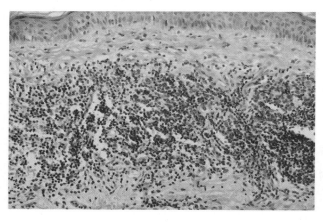

FIG. 29-27

Halo nevus. At low magnification a dense lymphocytic infiltrate is present without any obvious nevus cells. ($\times$ 64)

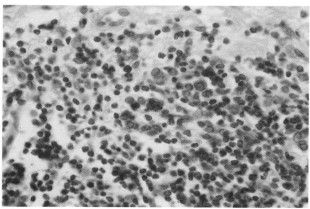

FIG. 29-28

Halo nevus, higher magnification of Fig. 29-27. The nevus has been almost completely destroyed. Only a few melanocytes are scattered throughout the lymphocytic infiltrate. ($\times$ 160)

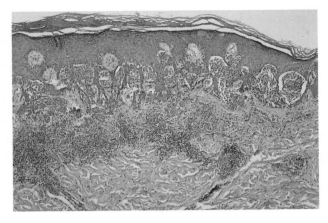

FIG. 29-29

Compound Spitz nevus. At the dermal-epidermal junction nevus cell nests are seen that show artifactual clefts between the nevus cell nests and the epidermis. (× 16)

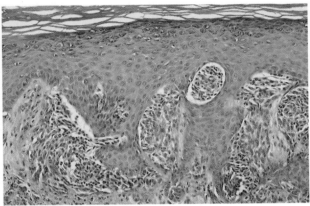

FIG. 29-30

Compound Spitz nevus. The nevus cells consist of spindle cells. The epidermis is hyperplastic and shows elongated rete ridges. (× 40)

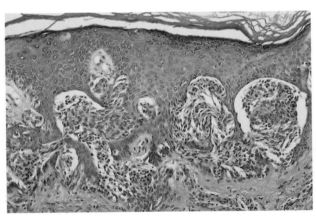

FIG. 29-31

Compound Spitz nevus. There are artifactual clefts above the nests of nevus cells at the dermal-epidermal junction. Part of the spindle-shaped nevus cells are arranged in whorls. (× 40)

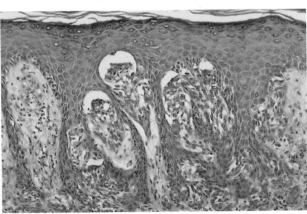

FIG. 29-32

Compound Spitz nevus. Melanin is, in many instances, completely or nearly completely absent in Spitz nevi. (× 40)

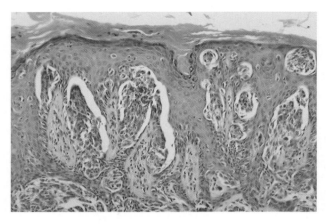

FIG. 29-33

Compound Spitz nevus. Artifactual clefts are seen between the nevus cell nests and the epidermis. Slight permeation of the epidermis by individual melanocytes and small nests of melanocytes are seen. (× 40)

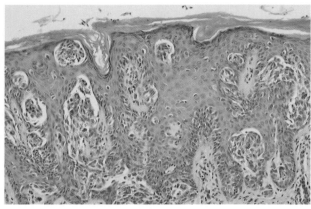

FIG. 29-34

Compound Spitz nevus. The epidermis is hyperplastic. Sharply demarcated nests with artifactual clefts between the cells and keratinocytes are present. (× 40)

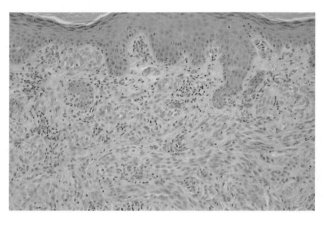

FIG. 29-35

Compound Spitz nevus. Most of the nevus cell nests are present in the dermis. They are spindle-shaped. (× 40)

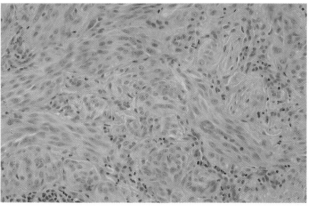

FIG. 29-36

Compound Spitz nevus. The spindle-shaped nevus cells do not contain any pigment. They are rather uniform in size and shape. (× 64)

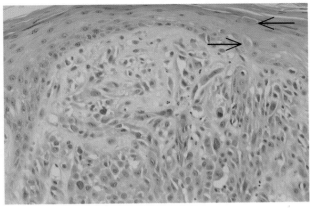

FIG. 29-37

Intradermal Spitz nevus. Within the overlying epidermis reddish globules resembling colloid bodies can be seen (arrows). In this Spitz nevus epithelioid cells predominate. The nevus cells are amelanotic. (× 64)

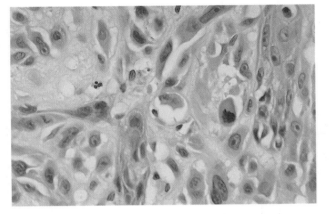

FIG. 29-38

Intradermal Spitz nevus, epithelioid cells predominating. The tumor cells vary in size and shape, and they are irregularly shaped. They have an eosinophilic cytoplasm. (× 160)

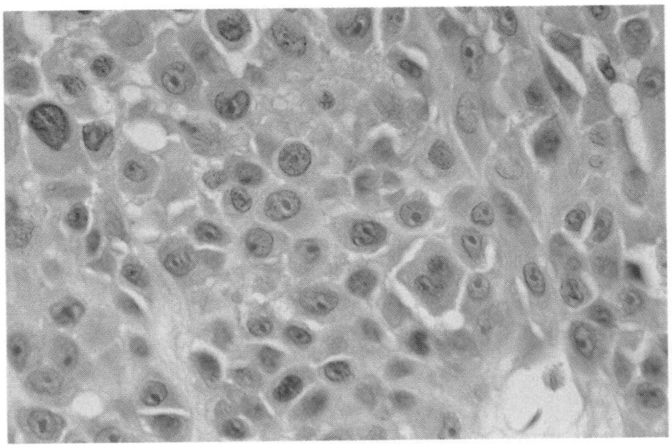

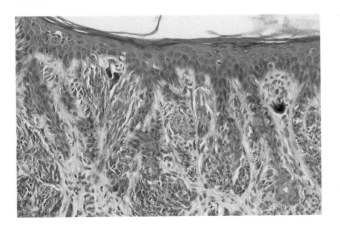

FIG. 29-39

Intradermal Spitz nevus. The epithelioid cells are large, polygonal, and sharply demarcated. They can be multinucleated. Melanin is absent. (× 160)

FIG. 29-40

Pigmented spindle cell nevus (Reed). At the dermal-epidermal junction spindle-shaped nevus cell nests are present, which are heavily pigmented. (× 64)

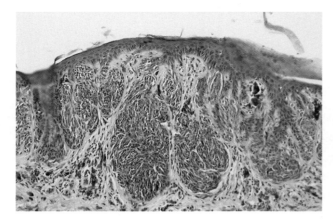

FIG. 29-41

Pigmented spindle cell nevus (Reed). The junctional spindle-shaped cells are arranged in nests and contain melanin in an even distribution. In contrast to a Spitz nevus, the nevus cell nests in this specimen do not show an artifactual cleft between nevus cells and epidermis. (× 40)

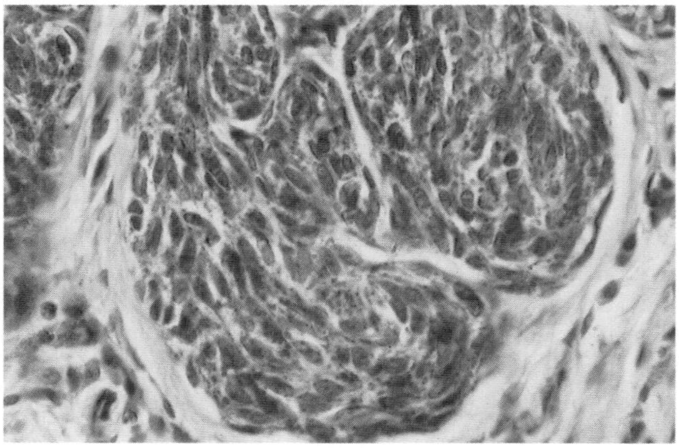

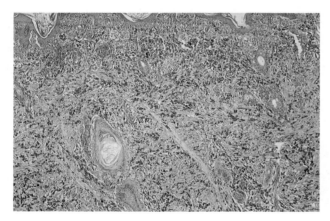

FIG. 29-42

Pigmented spindle-cell nevus (Reed), higher magnification of Fig. 29-41. The nevus cells have elongated nuclei and even distribution of melanin within the cytoplasm. (× 160)

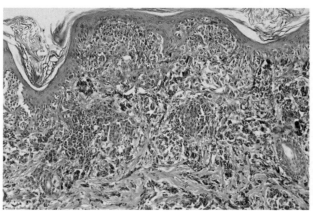

FIG. 29-43

Congenital nevus. Appearance in a newborn. At the dermal-epidermal junction and in the upper dermis nevus cells are present. In the lower dermis the melanocytes are scattered throughout. (× 16)

FIG. 29-44

Congenital nevus. Appearance in a newborn. At the dermal-epidermal junction nevus cell nests can be seen. Within the dermis nevus cells are present in well-defined nests as well as scattered throughout the dermis. (× 40)

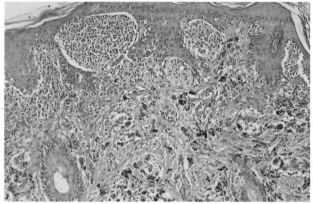

FIG. 29-45

Congenital nevus. Appearance in a newborn. The epidermis shows typical nevus cell nests as well as individual melanocytes scattered throughout the epidermis, simulating upward migration as seen in a superficial spreading malignant melanoma. ($\times$ 40)

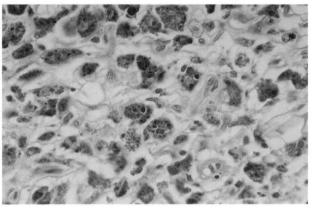

FIG. 29-46

Congenital nevus. Appearance in a newborn. The nevus cell nests contain melanin evenly distributed throughout the cytoplasm. ($\times$ 160)

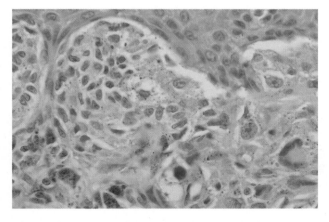

FIG. 29-47

Congenital nevus. Appearance in a newborn. Within the dermis the majority of nevus cells are scattered individually rather than occurring in nests. ($\times$ 160)

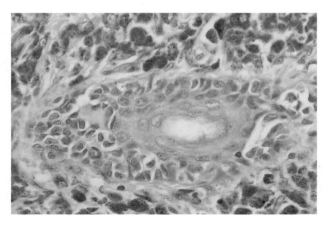

FIG. 29-48

Congenital nevus. Appearance in a newborn. In congenital nevi nevus cell nests may be found in adnexal structures, *i.e.,* in hair follicles, as on this picture. ($\times$ 160)

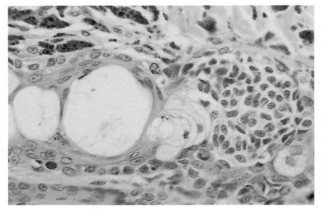

FIG. 29-49

Congenital nevus. Nevus cell nests are present in a sebaceous gland. (× 160)

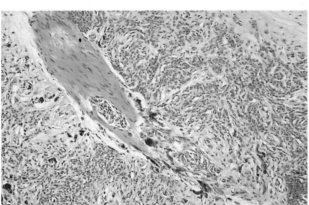

FIG. 29-50

Congenital nevus. Nevus cell nests are present in the dermis and in an arrector pili muscle. (× 40)

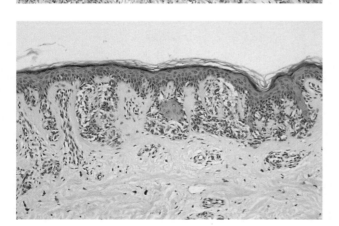

FIG. 29-51

Lentigo simplex with a junction nevus. The rete ridges show moderate elongation. Nevus cell nests are present at the epidermal–dermal junction. (× 40)

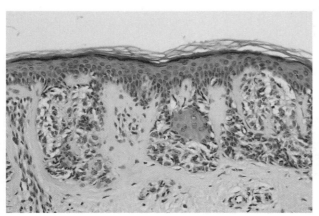

FIG. 29-52

Lentigo simplex with a junction nevus, higher magnification of Fig. 29-51. The rete ridges are elongated, nevus cell nests are seen at the epidermal–dermal junction. (× 64)

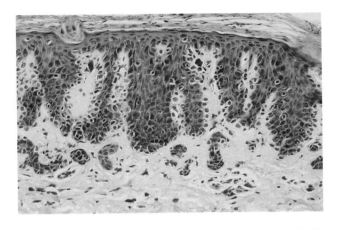

FIG. 29-53

Lengito simplex. The epidermis shows an elongation of the rete ridges, which are hyperpigmented and show an increased number of melanocytes. (× 64)

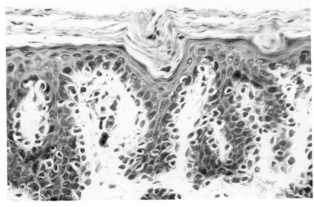

FIG. 29-54

Lentigo simplex. The elongated rete ridges are hyperpigmented and show an increased number of melanocytes. Melanophages are found in the dermis. (× 100)

Lichen planus like keratosis.

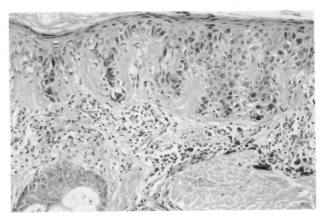

FIG. 29-55

Solar lentigo (lentigo senilis). The rete ridges are elongtaed and show small budlike extensions. The number of melanocytes is increased. The epidermis is hyperpigmented. (× 64)

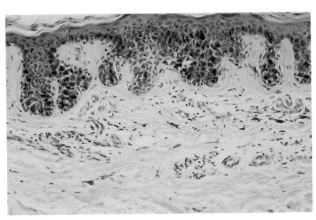

FIG. 29-56

Solar lentigo (lentigo senilis). The rete ridges appear club-shaped and show small budlike extensions. The rete ridges are composed of deeply pigmented basaloid cells intermingled with melanocytes. (× 64)

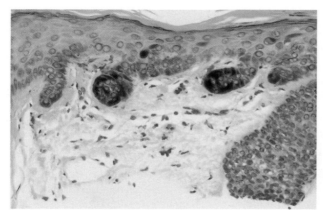

FIG. 29-57

Solar lentigo (lentigo senilis). The rete ridges are club-shaped and show considerable hyperpigmentation of the basal cells. (× 64)

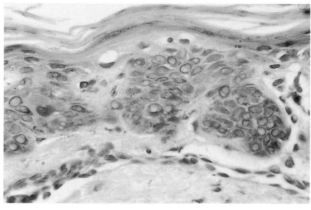

FIG. 29-58

Solar lentigo (lentigo senilis). The club-shaped rete ridges are hyperpigmented even though the melanocytes are not increased in number. (× 160)

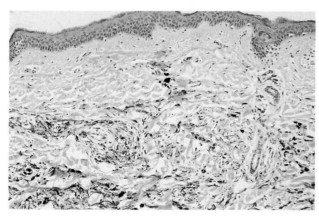

FIG. 29-59

Blue nevus, common type. Melanocytes lie grouped in irregular bundles in the dermis. The melanocytes have elongated dendritic processes. (× 40)

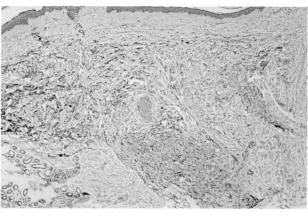

FIG. 29-60

Blue nevus, common type. Heavily pigmented dendritic melanocytes are arranged in bundles throughout the dermis. (× 16)

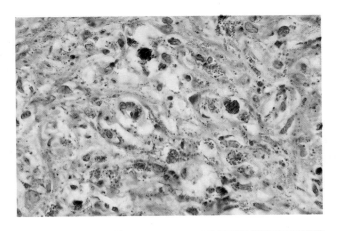

FIG. 29-61

Blue nevus, common type. The melanocytes are heavily pigmented. They are elongated, slender, and have long dendritic processes. They are not arranged in nests. (× 160)

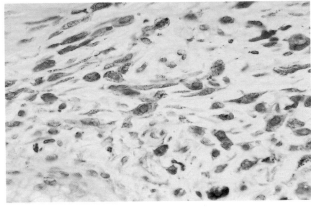

FIG. 29-62

Blue nevus, common type. The melanocytes have long, slender dendritic processes that are filled with fine melanin granules. In addition, melanophages are present with coarse and no dendritic processes. (× 160)

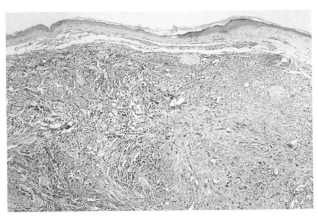

FIG. 29-63

Blue nevus, common type. Heavily pigmented melanocytes are grouped in irregular bundles in the lower dermis. (× 16)

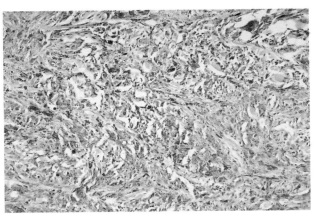

FIG. 29-64

Blue nevus, common type. The melanocytes have long dendritic processes that are filled with fine granules of melanin. (× 40)

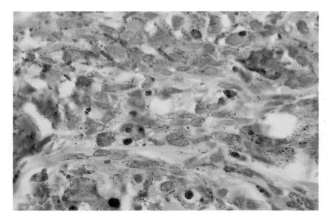

FIG. 29-65

Blue nevus, common type. The melanocytes are arranged in irregular bundles. They have elongated dendritic processes filled with melanin. Between the melanocytes some collagen is present. (× 240)

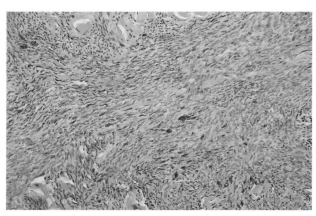

FIG. 29-66

Blue nevus, common type. The melanocytes contain fine melanin granules in an even distribution. (× 240)

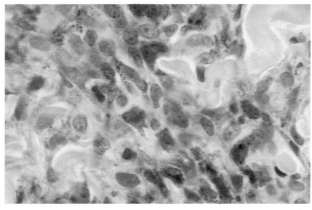

FIG. 29-67

Blue nevus, cellular type. Closely aggregated spindle-shaped melanocytes containing moderate amounts of melanin are present. The islands of spindle-shaped cells extend in various directions, and thus resemble the storiform pattern seen in a neurofibroma. (× 40)

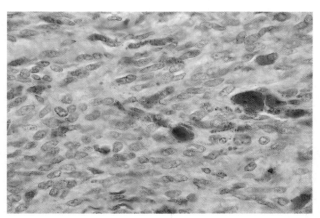

FIG. 29-68

Blue nevus, cellular type. The melanocytes appear spindle-shaped or rounded, depending on the angle at which they are sectioned. (× 160)

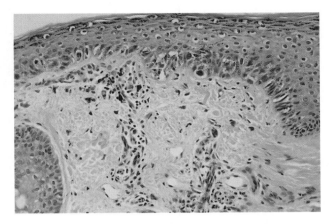

FIG. 29·69

Lentigo maligna. The basal melanocytes are increased in number, have hyperchromatic nuclei, and are hyperpigmented. (× 64)

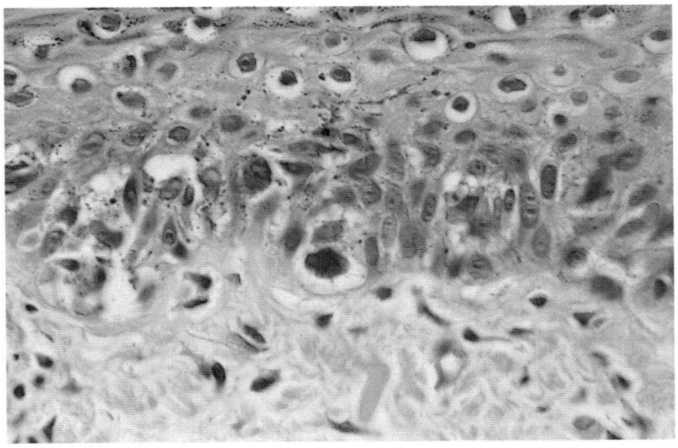

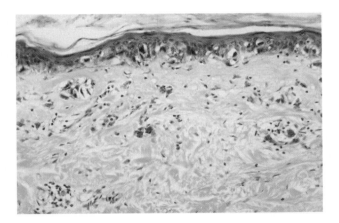

FIG. 29·70

Lentigo maligna, higher magnification of Fig. 29-69. The basal cell layer is hyperpigmented, and the epidermis shows an increased number of melanocytes and some irregularity in their arrangement. (× 160)

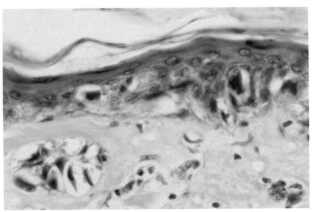

FIG. 29·71

Lentigo maligna melanoma. The epidermis is atrophic. The basal melanocytes show a marked increase in concentration. One nest of atypical melanocytes is seen in the dermis. (× 40)

FIG. 29·72

Lentigo maligna melanoma. The basal melanocytes are increased in number, appear pleomorphic and contain a considerable amount of melanin. Invasion is seen on the left side consisting of a nest of atypical melanocytes. (× 100)

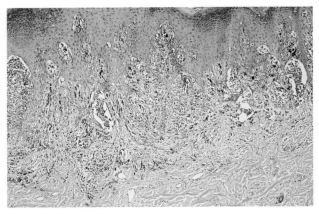

FIG. 29-73

Acral lentiginous melanoma in situ. The epidermis shows acanthosis and nests of hyperpigmented atypical melanocytes in the lower epidermis. Rounded, pagetoid melanocytes are seen in the upper epidermis. (× 16)

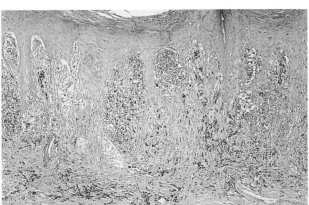

FIG. 29-74

Acral lentiginous melanoma in situ. The epidermis shows acanthosis and considerable hyperpigmentation. Atypical melanocytes are arranged in nests in the lower epidermis. (× 16)

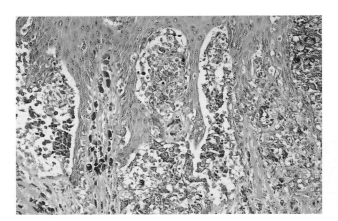

FIG. 29-75

Acral lentiginous melanoma in situ. The melanocytes are hyperpigmented and several melanocytes show hyperchromatic nuclei. Melanophages are present in the dermal papillae. (× 40)

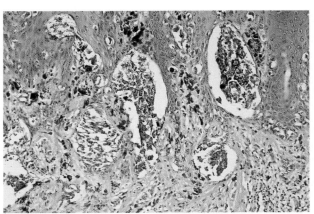

FIG. 29-76

Acral lentiginous melanoma in situ. Some of the melanocytes are spindle-shaped, especially in the lower epidermis, whereas other melanocytes, especially in the upper epidermis, are rounded and pagetoid. (× 40)

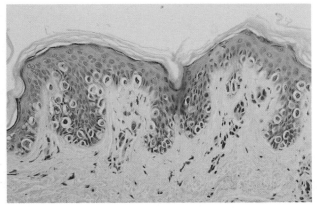

FIG. 29-77

Superficial spreading melanoma in situ. Rather uniformly rounded, large melanocytes are scattered in the lower epidermis. (× 64)

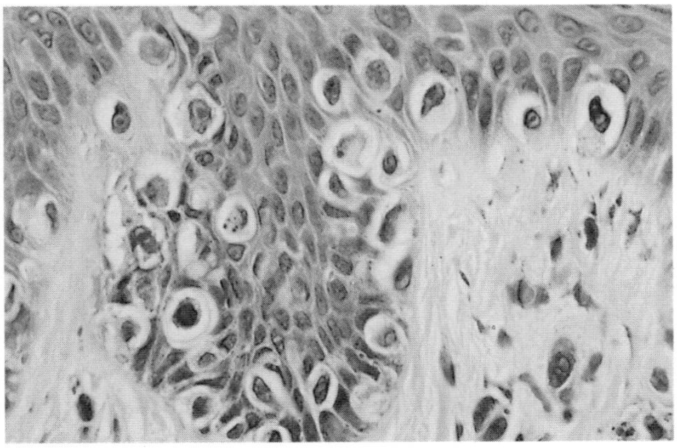

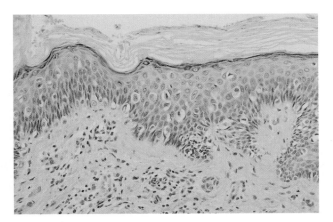

FIG. 29-78

Superficial spreading melanoma in situ, higher magnification of Fig. 29-77. The atypical melanocytes are round and large, and several show hyperchromatic nuclei. (× 160)

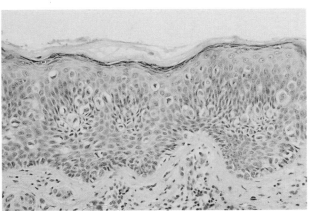

FIG. 29-79

Superficial spreading melanoma in situ. Atypical melanocytes with hyperchromatic nuclei are scattered in a pagetoid pattern throughout the epidermis. (× 64)

FIG. 29-80

Superficial spreading melanoma in situ. Rounded, large melanocytes with atypical, hyperchromatic nuclei are scattered throughout the epidermis. (× 64)

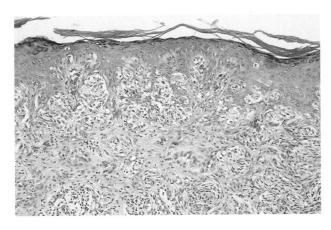

FIG. 29-81

Superficial spreading melanoma. At the dermal-epidermal junction and within the dermis nests of atypical melanocytes are seen. There is upward extension of tumor cells within the epidermis. (× 40)

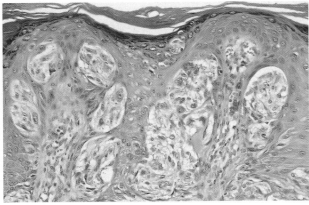

FIG. 29-82

Superficial spreading melanoma. Some of the atypical melanocytes are epithelioid; others are spindle-shaped. There is upward migration of atypical melanocytes singly and in small nests. (× 64)

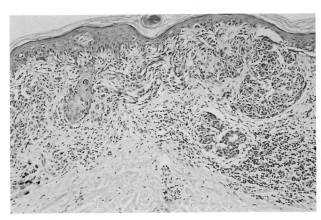

FIG. 29-83

Superficial spreading melanoma. At the dermal-epidermal junction and in the dermis nests of atypical spindle-shaped melanocytes are seen. A few pagetoid melanocytes are present in the upper epidermis. The melanocytes in the dermal nests do not show a decrease in size (absence of "maturation"). (× 40)

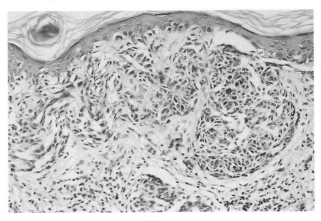

FIG. 29-84

Superficial spreading melanoma, higher magnification of Fig. 29-83. The melanocytes are irregular in shape, have hyperchromatic nuclei, and show lack of maturation in the deeper dermis. (× 64)

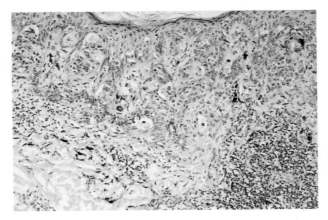

FIG. 29-85

Superficial spreading melanoma. There is considerable irregular junctional activity. The epidermis shows irregular downward proliferations of its rete ridges. Upward migration of melanoma cells is seen in the epidermis. On the right side of the photomicrograph, an inflammatory infiltrate is present. (× 40)

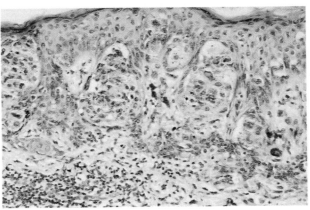

FIG. 29-86

Superficial spreading melanoma, higher magnification of Fig. 29-85. The melanocytes have atypical nuclei and contain melanin in an uneven distribution. An inflammatory infiltrate is present underneath the tumor. (× 64)

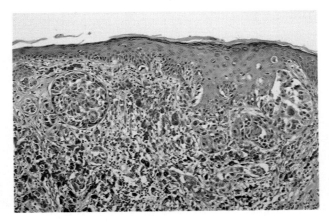

FIG. 29-87

Superficial spreading melanoma. The epidermis shows irregular junctional activity and upward migration of single melanocytes. There is a considerable number of melanophages between the dermal nests of atypical melanocytes. (× 40)

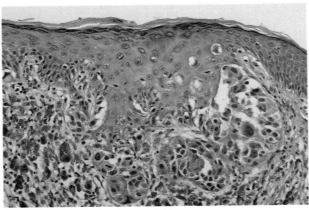

FIG. 29-88

Superficial spreading melanoma, higher magnification of Fig. 29-87. There is upward migration of atypical melanocytes. The atypical melanocytes at the dermal-epidermal junction are of the epithelioid cell type. (× 64)

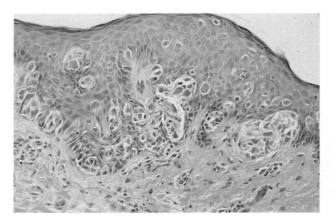

FIG. 29-89

Superficial spreading melanoma. The epidermis is permeated by nests of atypical melanocytes that have large nuclei. (× 64)

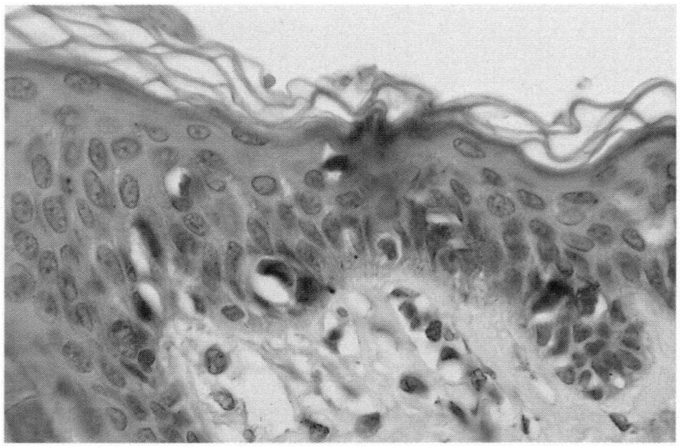

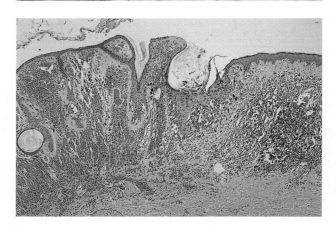

FIG. 29-90

Superficial spreading melanoma, edge of a lesion, incubation with a monoclonal antibody against melanoma cells. The nuclei of the atypical melanocytes are hyperchromatic. The melanocytes show upward migration. APAAP technique. (× 240)

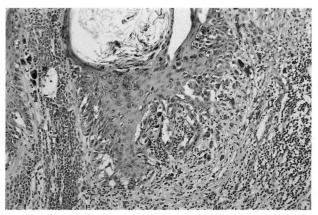

FIG. 29-91

Superficial spreading melanoma arising in a compound nevus. The compound nevus is seen on the left, the melanoma in the middle. On the right side of the photomicrograph an inflammatory infiltrate is seen. (× 16)

FIG. 29-92

Superficial spreading melanoma arising in a compound nevus. Nevus cell nests are seen on the left side. The melanoma is present in the center of the picture. It consists of irregular junctional activity with upward migration of atypical melanocytes. The stratum corneum is hyperpigmented. On the right side of the photomicrograph a lymphocytic infiltrate is seen. (× 40)

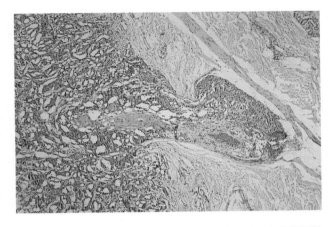

FIG. 29-93
Superficial spreading melanoma spreading down a hair follicle. The outer root sheath of the hair follicle has been replaced by melanoma cells. ($\times$ 16)

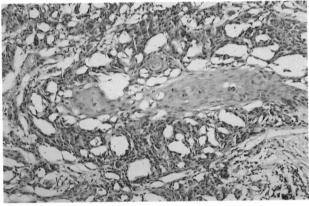

FIG. 29-94
Superficial spreading melanoma spreading down a hair follicle. The outer root sheath has been replaced almost entirely by melanoma cells. ($\times$ 40)

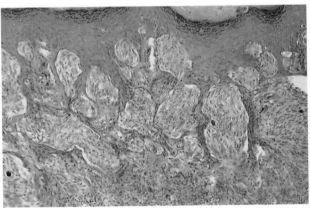

FIG. 29-95
Superficial spreading melanoma, spindle cell type. At the dermal-epidermal junction and in the upper dermis nests of atypical spindle-shaped melanocytes are present. ($\times$ 40)

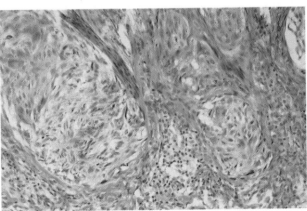

FIG. 29-96
Superficial spreading melanoma, spindle cell type. The tumor cells are spindle-shaped and lie in irregularly branching formations. ($\times$ 64)

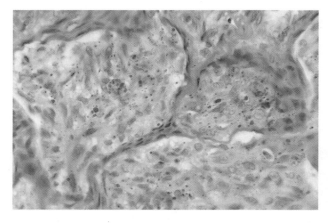

FIG. 29-97

Superficial spreading melanoma, spindle cell type. The tumor cells possess atypical nuclei and contain varying amounts of melanin. (× 160)

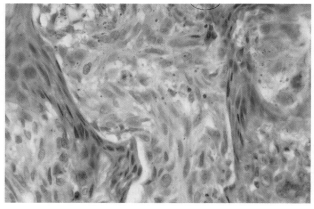

FIG. 29-98

Superficial spreading melanoma, spindle cell type. The nuclei of the tumor cells vary in size and shape. (× 160)

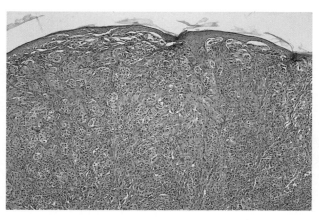

FIG. 29-99

Nodular malignant melanoma. The tumor cells have spread vertically down into the dermis. No upward migration of melanocytes is present in the epidermis. (× 16)

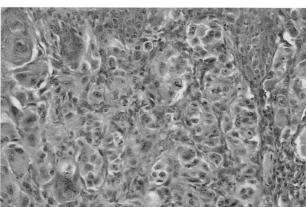

FIG. 29-100

Nodular malignant melanoma. The atypical melanocytes are of the epithelioid cell type and are arranged in alveolar formations. A mitotic figure is present in the center of the picture. (× 64)

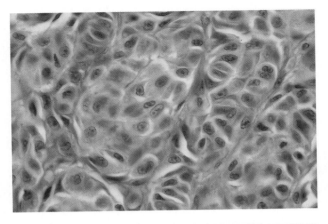

FIG. 29·101
Nodular malignant melanoma, higher magnification of Fig. 29-100. The tumor cells are epithelioid type of cells arranged in alveolar formations. (× 160)

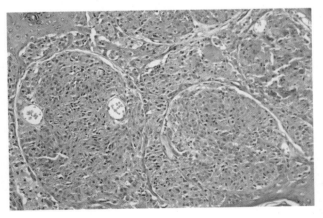

FIG. 29·102
Nodular malignant melanoma, higher magnification of Fig. 29-100. The tumor cells have large nuclei and can be multinucleated. (× 160)

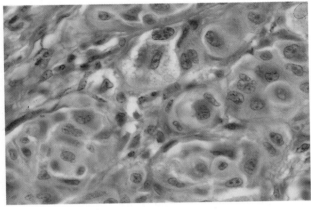

FIG. 29·103
Nodular malignant melanoma. Pigmented nests of atypical melanocytes are present in the dermis. (× 40)

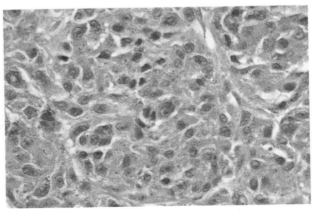

FIG. 29·104
Nodular malignant melanoma. Epithelioid type of cells are present that contain a considerable amount of melanin. (× 160)

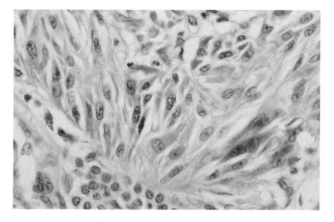

FIG. 29-105

Nodular malignant melanoma, spindle cell type. The nevus cell nests show pleomorphic nuclei. (× 160)

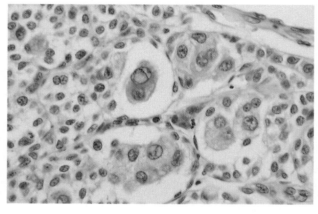

FIG. 29-106

Nodular malignant melanoma. Atypical multinucleated melanocytes are present. (× 160)

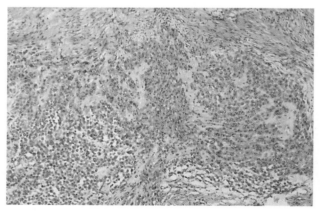

FIG. 29-107

Nodular malignant melanoma arising in a bathing trunk congenital nevus. The melanoma has arisen deep in the dermis and largely consists of undifferentiated cells. (× 16)

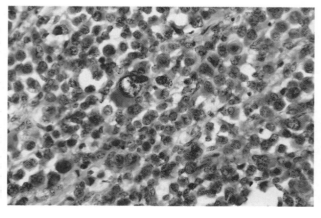

FIG. 29-108

Nodular malignant melanoma arising in a bathing trunk congenital nevus. The undifferentiated cells resemble lymphoblasts. They do not contain melanin, but showed a positive reaction when incubated with antibody against S 100 protein. (× 100)

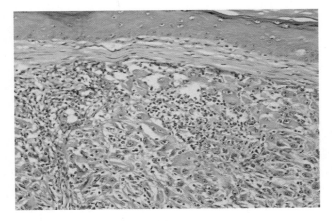

FIG. 29-109

Nodular malignant melanoma resembling a fibroxanthoma. Within the dermis large atypical cells with abundant cytoplasm are seen. This section does not show junctional activity, but when serial sections were performed, junctional activity was seen. (× 40)

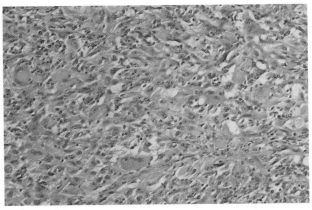

FIG. 29-110

Nodular malignant melanoma resembling a fibroxanthoma. The atypical melanocytes have abundant cytoplasm and stain eosinophilic. (× 40)

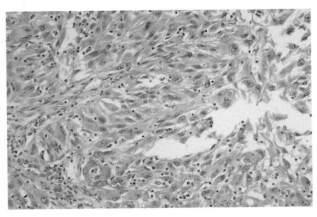

FIG. 29-111

Nodular malignant melanoma resembling a fibroxanthoma. Incubation with an antibody against S 100 protein reveals a positive reaction. ABC technique. (× 64)

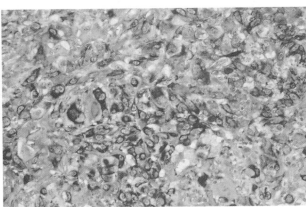

FIG. 29-112

Nodular malignant melanoma resembling a fibroxanthoma. Incubation with a monoclonal antibody against vimentin reveals a positive reaction. This reaction would be positive also in a fibroxanthoma. APAAP technique. (× 40)

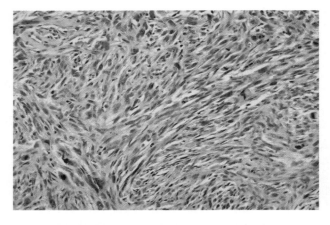

FIG. 29-113

Nodular spindle cell malignant melanoma resembling a fibrosarcoma. The tumor consists of branching bundles of atypical spindle cells. (× 64)

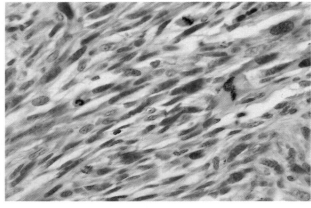

FIG. 29-114

Nodular spindle cell malignant melanoma resembling a fibrosarcoma, higher magnification. Several mitoses are present. The nuclei are elongated, large, and hyperchromatic. (× 160)

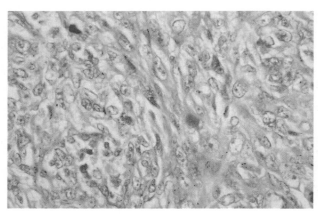

FIG. 29-115

Nodular spindle cell malignant melanoma resembling a fibrosarcoma, Fontana-Masson stain for the demonstration of melanin. The lesion is amelanotic. (× 160)

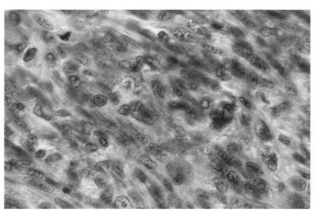

FIG. 29-116

Nodular spindle cell malignant melanoma resembling a fibrosarcoma. Incubation with an antibody against S 100 protein revels a positive reaction. This reaction would be negative in a fibrosarcoma. ABC technique. (× 160)

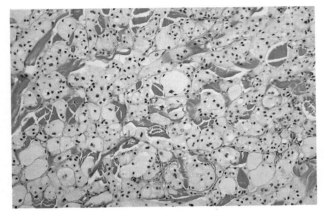

FIG. 29-117

Balloon cell malignant melanoma. This melanoma consists of balloon cells with a varying number of atypical melanocytes. (× 40)

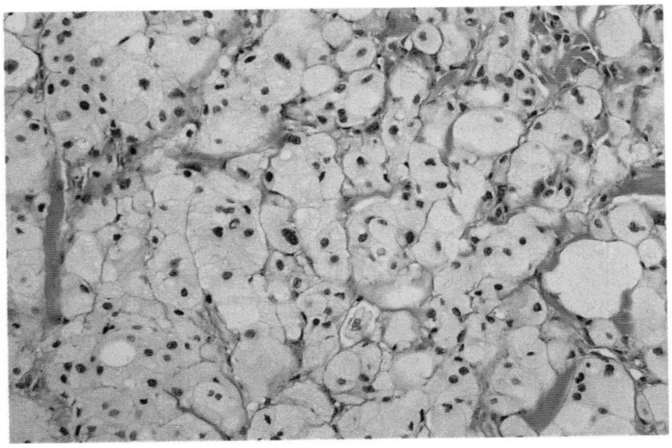

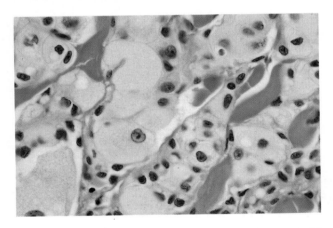

FIG. 29-118

Balloon cell malignant melanoma. Several balloon cells have large hyperchromatic nuclei. (× 64)

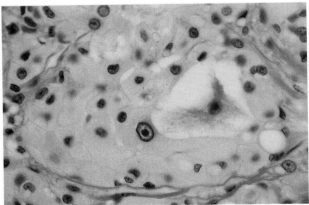

FIG. 29-119

Balloon cell malignant melanoma. The balloon cells vary in size and shape. (× 160)

FIG. 29-120

Balloon cell malignant melanoma. The balloon cells show nuclear atypia. (× 160)

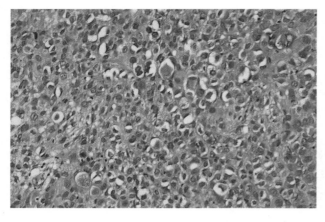

FIG. 29-121

Metastasis of a malignant melanoma. The cells look atypical and are amelanotic. Without special stains, it is impossible to identify them as melanoma cells. (× 64)

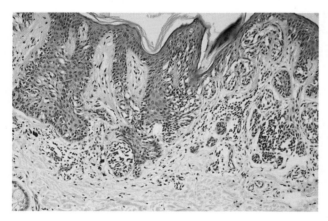

FIG. 29-122

Metastasis of a malignant melanoma. Incubation with an antibody against S 100 protein helps to identify the cells as melanoma cells. PAP technique. (× 64)

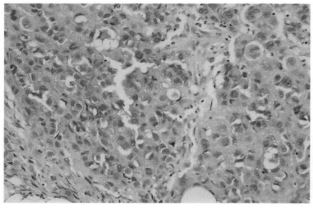

FIG. 29-123

Dysplastic nevus, lentiginous type. The rete ridges are elongated and show irregularly scattered melanocytes. The cytoplasm of the melanocytes has retracted around the nuclei, which most likely is an artifact. (× 40)

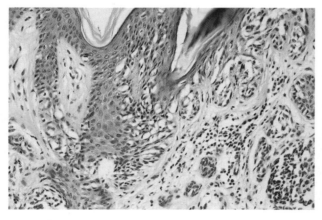

FIG. 29-124

Dysplastic nevus, lentiginous type, higher magnification of Fig. 29-123. The basal cells have been replaced by melanocytes in many areas. The melanocytes show an irregular distribution and may be arranged in small groups, but do not form typical nests. (× 64)

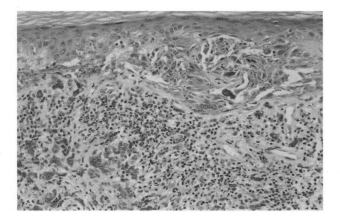

FIG. 29-125

Dysplastic junction nevus. The nevus cell nests consist of spindle cell melanocytes with their long axis arranged parallel to the epidermis. An inflammatory infiltrate containing melanophages is present in the upper dermis. (× 64)

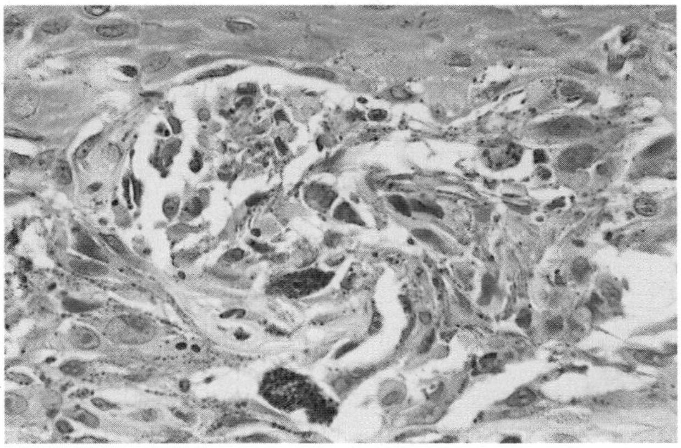

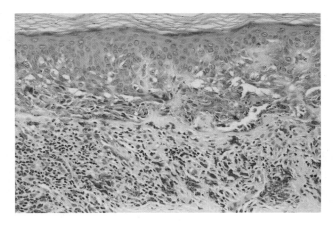

FIG. 29-126

Dysplastic junction nevus, higher magnification of Fig. 29-125. Several melanocytes have hyperchromatic atypical-appearing nuclei with melanin distributed throughout the cytoplasm. (× 160)

FIG. 29-127

Dysplastic junction nevus. Atypical-appearing melanocytes in the junctional nests are spindle-shaped and lie parallel to the dermal-epidermal interface. (× 64)

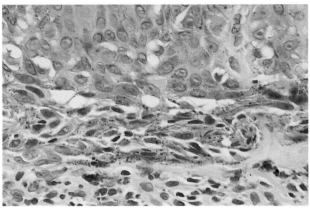

FIG. 29-128

Dysplastic junction nevus, higher magnification of Fig. 29-127. The spindle-shaped melanocytes are arranged with their long axis parallel to the epidermis. They contain melanin in a fine, dusty distribution. (× 160)

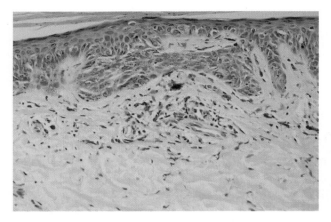

FIG. 29-129

Dysplastic junction nevus. The melanocytes at the dermal-epidermal junction are irregularly shaped and extend with their long axis parallel to the epidermis. ($\times$ 64)

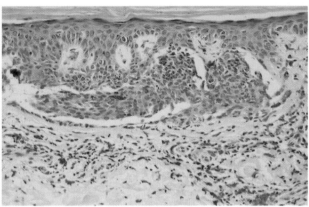

FIG. 29-130

Dysplastic junction nevus. The spindle cell melanocytes are arranged parallel to the epidermis and connect several rete ridges. The dermis shows an inflammatory infiltrate consisting of lymphoid cells. ($\times$ 64)

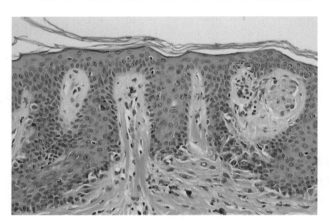

FIG. 29-131

Dysplastic junction nevus. Spindle cell melanocytes are arranged in nests at the dermal-epidermal junction with their long axis parallel to the epidermis. ($\times$ 64)

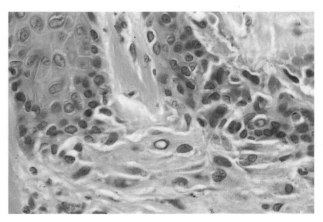

FIG. 29-132

Dysplastic junction nevus, higher magnification of Fig. 29-131. The melanocytes have hyperchromatic nuclei and extend from one rete ridge to the next. ($\times$ 160)

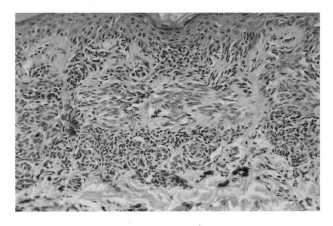

FIG. 29-133

Dysplastic compound nevus. Spindle-shaped cells are present in the papillary dermis and extend with their long axis parallel to the epidermis. The melanocytes in the nests beneath the spindle-shaped cells look much more uniform and show good maturation. (× 64)

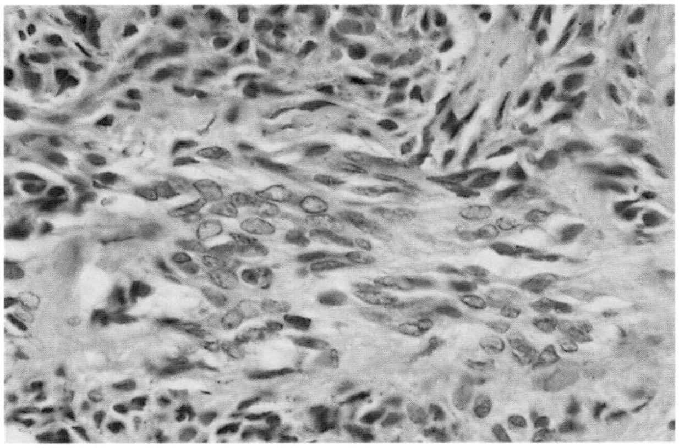

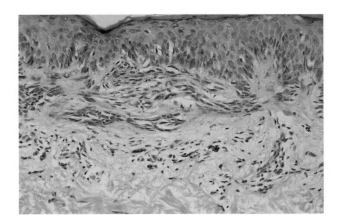

FIG. 29-134

Dysplastic compound nevus, higher magnification of Fig. 29-133. The nevus cells are spindle-shaped and arranged with their long axis parallel to the epidermis. (× 160)

FIG. 29-135

Dysplastic compound nevus. Spindle-shaped nevus cell nests are present at the dermal-epidermal junction and in the upper dermis. (× 64)

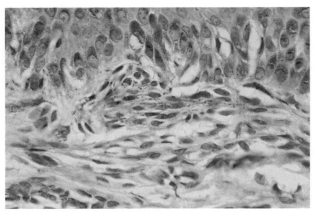

FIG. 29-136

Dysplastic compound nevus, higher magnification of Fig. 29-135. The spindle cells contain melanin in a fine, dusty distribution. (× 160)

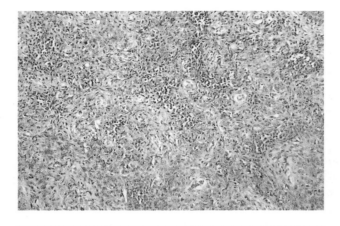

FIG. 29-137

Malignant blue nevus. At low magnification the lesion looks like a cellular blue nevus with varying amounts of melanin. (× 40)

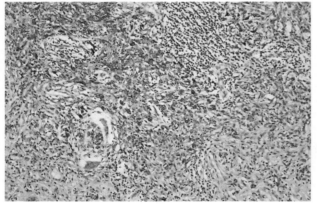

FIG. 29-138

Malignant blue nevus, higher magnification of Fig. 29-137. In the lower portion of the photomicrograph atypical multinucleated melanocytes are present. (× 64)

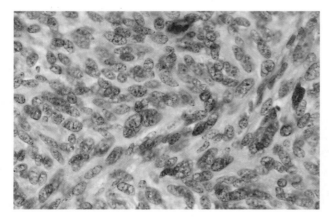

FIG. 29-139

Malignant blue nevus. Higher magnification shows that the atypical nuclei vary in size and shape. Melanin is present in several tumor cells and lies within branching dendritic processes. (× 160)

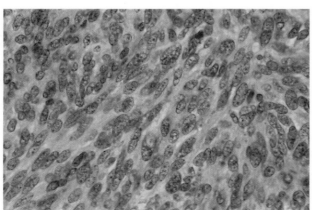

FIG. 29-140

Malignant blue nevus. The tumor contains anaplastic nuclei, some of which are elongated. Several tumor cells contain melanin in dendritic processes. (× 160)

CHAPTER 30

Lymphoma

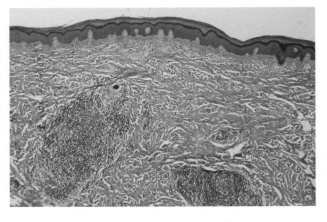

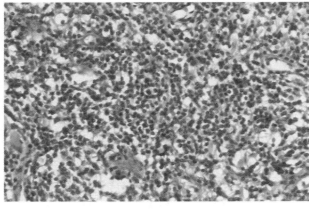

FIG. 30-1

Small-cell lymphoma (lymphocytic lymphoma, well-differentiated lymphoma). In the dermis two well-circumscribed masses of lymphoctyes can be seen. (× 16)

FIG. 30-2

Small-cell lymphoma (lymphocytic lymphoma, well-differentiated lymphoma), higher magnification of Fig. 30-1. The predominant cell is the small lymphocyte. (× 64)

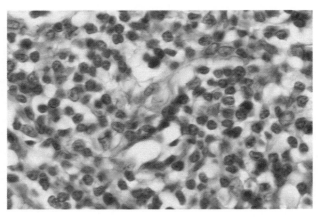

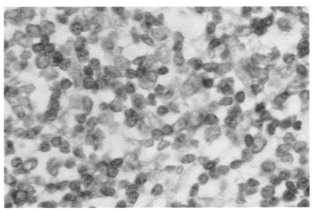

FIG. 30-3

Small-cell lymphoma (lymphocytic lymphoma, well-differentiated lymphoma). The lymphocytes have a round nucleus and hardly any visible cytoplasm. An occasional large lymphocyte is mixed in. (× 160)

FIG. 30-4

Small-cell lymphoma (lymphocytic lymphoma, well-differentiated lymphoma), Giemsa stain. The predominant cell is the small lymphocyte with a round nucleus. (× 160) The diagnosis of malignant lymphoma in Fig. 30-1 through Fig. 30-4 is based on clinical data.

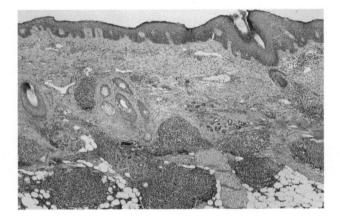

FIG. 30-5

Mixed small- and large-cell lymphocytic lymphoma. Masses of densely packed tumor cells are present in the lower dermis and subcutaneous fat. (× 16)

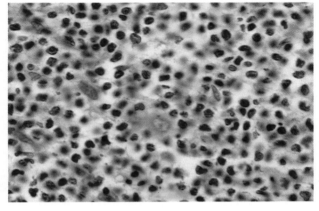

FIG. 30-6

Mixed small- and large-cell lymphocytic lymphoma, higher magnification of Fig. 30-5. Two cell populations are present: (1) cells with small, dark nuclei, representing well-differentiated lymphocytes, and (2) cells with large, pale-staining nuclei, representing a centroblast or immunoblast. (× 64)

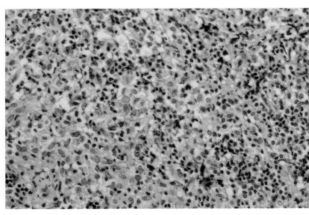

FIG. 30-7

Mixed small- and large-cell lymphocytic lymphoma. The tumor consists of small lymphocytes with a dark nucleus and large lymphocytes with a pale-staining nucleus. (× 64)

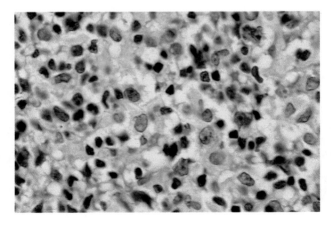

FIG. 30-8

Mixed small- and large-cell lymphocytic lymphoma, higher magnification of Fig. 30-7. The small lymphocytes have dark nuclei with hardly any visible cytoplasm. The large lymphocytes have large, pale-staining nuclei with abundant cytoplasm. (× 160)

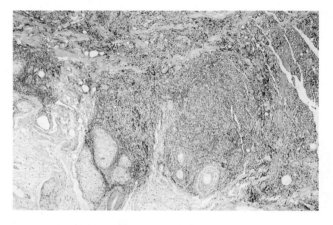

FIG. 30-9

Large-cell lymphoma (poorly differentiated lymphoma). At low magnification a diffuse infiltration of lymphocytes in the dermis is seen. (× 16)

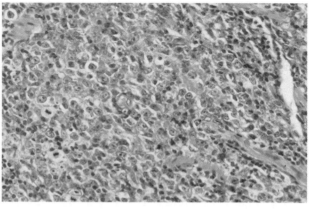

FIG. 30-10

Large-cell lymphoma (poorly differentiated lymphoma). The predominant cell type is a large lymphocyte with a pale-staining nucleus. (× 64)

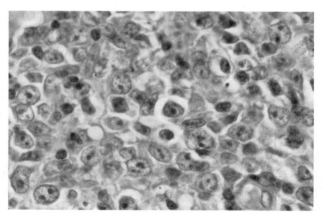

FIG. 30-11

Large-cell lymphoma (poorly differentiated lymphoma). The tumor predominantly shows immunoblasts with a few centroblasts mixed in. Immunoblasts have large, light nuclei with very large nucleoli. The latter are often solitary and located in the center of the nucleus. Centroblasts have a round nucleus. Several medium-sized nucleoli are often found at the inner nuclear membrane. (× 160)

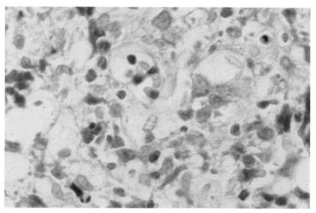

FIG. 30-12

Large-cell lymphoma (poorly differentiated lymphoma), Giemsa stain. The lymphocytes have large, pale-staining nuclei with a pale cytoplasm. (× 160)

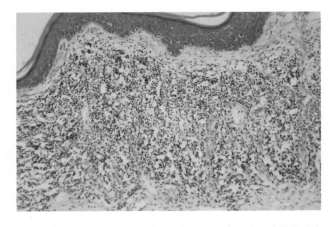

FIG. 30-13

Small T helper-cell lymphoma with low malignancy. Fig. 30-13 through Fig. 30-16 show the same tumor. A dense infiltration with small lymphocytes is present in the upper dermis. There is little epidermotropism. (× 40)

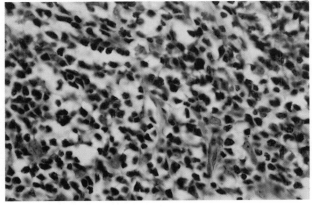

FIG. 30-14

Small T helper-cell lymphoma with low malignancy. The predominant cell is the small lymphocyte with a dark-staining nucleus. (× 160)

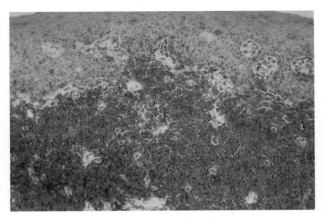

FIG. 30-15

Small T helper-cell lymphoma with low malignancy. Incubation with a monoclonal antibody against T helper cells (Leu 3a) shows uniform labeling of the lymphocytes in the dermis. Numerous Leu 3a-positive cells are also present in the epidermis. (× 40)

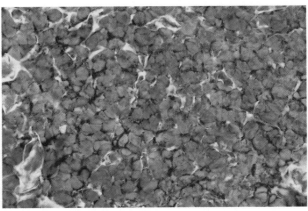

FIG. 30-16

Small T helper-cell lymphoma with low malignancy. Incubation with the monoclonal antibody Leu 3a against T helper cells, higher magnification of Fig. 30-15. Almost each cell is labeled. (× 160)

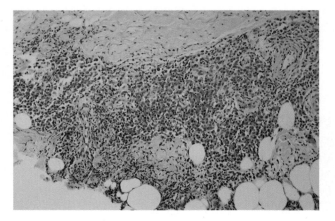

FIG. 30-17

Large T helper-cell lymphoma with high malignancy. Fig. 30-17 through Fig. 30-21 show the same tumor. At the junction of the dermis and subcutaneous fat a dense infiltrate of lymphocytic cells is seen. (× 40)

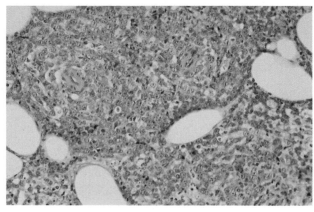

FIG. 30-18

Large T helper-cell lymphoma with high malignancy. The cells are large and show pale nuclei with dark nucleoli. They lie close together. (× 64)

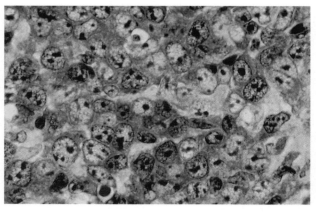

FIG. 30-19

Large T helper-cell lymphoma with high malignancy, Giemsa stain. The atypical or immature lymphocytes have prominent nucleoli (× 160)

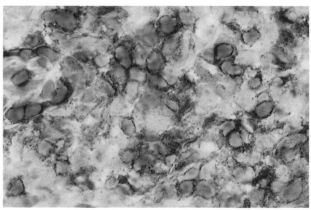

FIG. 30-20

Large T helper-cell lymphoma with high malignancy. Incubation with the monoclonal antibody Leu 3a, which reacts with T helper cells. The majority of cells are labeled. APAAP technique. (× 240)

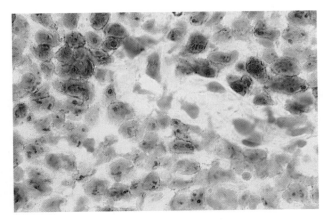

FIG. 30-21

Large T helper-cell lymphoma with high malignancy. Incubation with the anti-proliferation antibody Ki 67. The antibody shows a positive reaction with nuclei or nucleoli of cells undergoing mitosis. Thus, if many cells show a positive reaction, as in this lymphoma, the lymphoma is considered highly malignant. APAAP technique. (× 240)

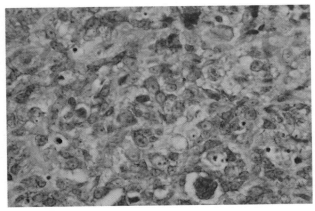

FIG. 30-22

Immunoblastic B cell lymphoma with high malignancy, Giemsa stain. Fig. 30-22 through Fig. 30-23 show the same tumor. The tumor consists of atypical pale-staining lymphocytes with large nucleoli. One giant cell is shown. (× 160)

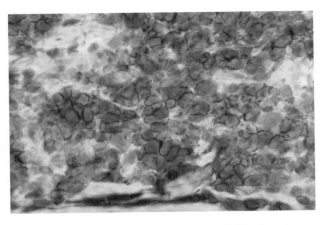

FIG. 30-23

Immunoblastic B cell lymphoma with high malignancy. Incubation with a monoclonal antibody against B cells. The majority of tumor cells show a positive reaction. At the bottom of the picture single-row invasion of lymphocytes can be seen. APAAP technique. (× 160)

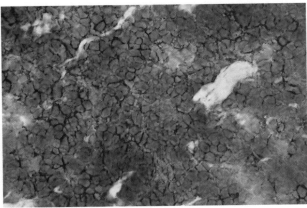

FIG. 30-24

B cell lymphoma. Incubation with a monoclonal antibody against B cells shows uniform labeling. (× 160)

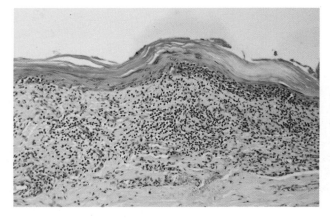

FIG. 30-25

Mycosis fungoides, early stage. The epidermis is flattened. Subepidermally a bandlike inflammatory infiltrate lying close to the epidermis is seen. The infiltrate invades the epidermis in some areas. The histologic picture resembles that of poikiloderma atrophicans vasculare. (× 40)
Fig 39-25 through Fig. 30-29 represent the same lesion.

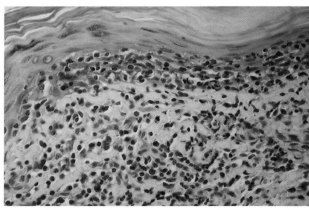

FIG. 30-26

Mycosis fungoides, early stage. Small collections of cells with hyperchromatic nuclei are present in the lower portion of the epidermis. Subepidermally a dense infiltrate of small lymphocytes is seen. (× 100)

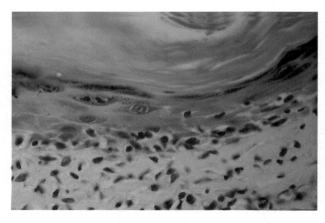

FIG. 30-27

Mycosis fungoides, early stage. Small groups or single lymphocytes have invaded the epidermis. The basal keratinocytes show hydropic degeneration; the epidermis is atrophic. The histologic picture resembles poikiloderma atrophicans vasculare. (× 100)

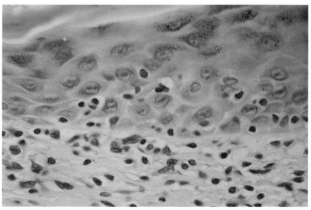

FIG. 30-28

Mycosis fungoides, early stage. In the epidermis the lymphocytes lie singly as "haloed" cells, but also in small clusters. (× 160)

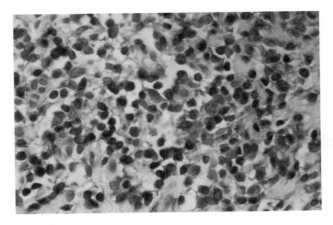

FIG. 30-29

Mycosis fungoides, early stage. Incubation of a paraffin section with a monoclonal antibody against T cells. Almost all cells in the infiltrate show a positive reaction. APAAP technique. (× 160)

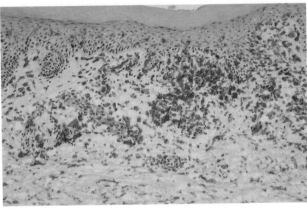

FIG. 30-30

Mycosis fungoides, early stage. Fig. 30-30 through Fig. 30-32 show the same tumor. Incubation with a monoclonal antibody against Langerhans cells (Leu 6) shows that Langerhans cells are greatly increased in number in mycosis fungoides. (× 40)

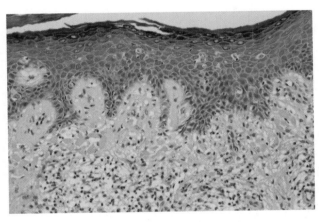

FIG. 30-31

Mycosis fungoides, early stage. The epidermis shows epidermotropism without spongiosis. (× 64)

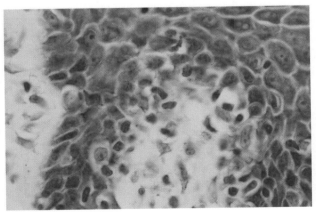

FIG. 30-32

Mycosis fungoides, early stage, Giemsa stain. On the right side small Pautrier abscesses are seen consisting of cells with hyperchromatic nuclei and cells with large, pale nuclei. Most likely the former are T helper and the latter Langerhans cells. (× 240)

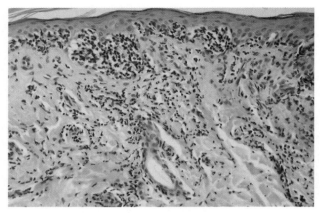

FIG. 30-33

Mycosis fungoides. Several Pautrier microabscesses are present in the lower portion of the epidermis. Pautrier microabscesses consist of small intraepidermal groups of tightly aggregated mononuclear cells located within a vacuole. (× 64)

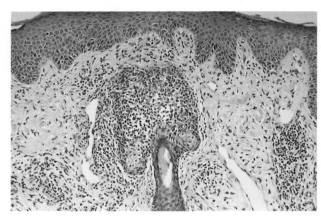

FIG. 30-34

Mycosis fungoides. Epidermotropism can also involve hair follicles, as in this photomicrograph that shows dense aggregates of lymphocytes. (× 40)

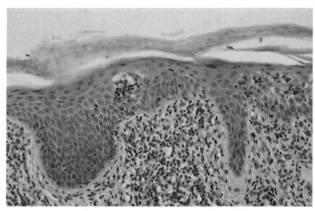

FIG. 30-35

Mycosis fungoides. The epidermis shows several Pautrier microabscesses. A dense lymphocytic infiltrate is present in the dermis. (× 64)

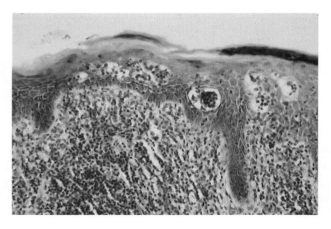

FIG. 30-36

Mycosis fungoides, Giemsa stain. The epidermis contains several Pautrier microabscesses. Subepidermally a dense lymphocytic infiltrate is present. (× 64)

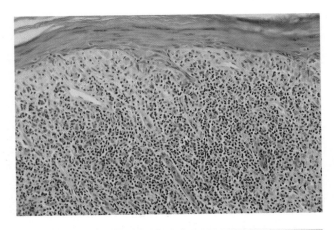

FIG. 30-37

Mycosis fungoides. A dense lymphocytic infiltrate is present in the dermis. The epidermis has become atrophic. (× 64)

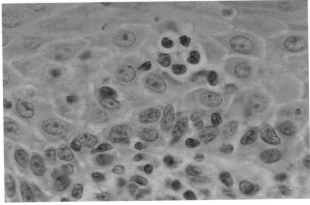

FIG. 30-38

Mycosis fungoides. The Pautrier microabscesses consist of Langerhans cells and lymphocytes with hyperchromatic convoluted nuclei. (× 160)

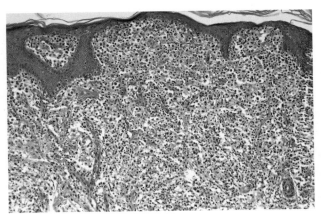

FIG. 30-39

Mycosis fungoides, tumor stage. The upper dermis contains a dense lymphocytic infiltrate that is bandlike. The infiltrate cells show hyperchromatic nuclei. This photomicrograph shows only slight epidermotropism. The infiltrate compresses the epidermis. (× 40)

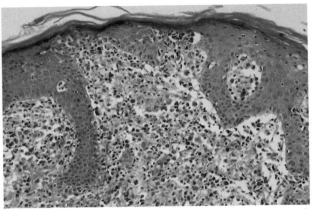

FIG. 30-40

Mycosis fungoides, tumor stage. The epidermis shows Pautrier microabscesses, and the dermis shows a dense infiltrate of lymphocytes with hyperchromatic, irregularly shaped "cerebriform" nuclei, representing mycosis cells. (× 64)

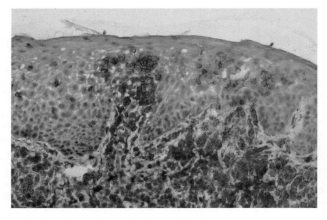

FIG. 30-41

Mycosis fungoides. Incubation with a monoclonal antibody against T helper cells (Leu 3a). The dermis shows a dense infiltrate of T helper cells, and the epidermis contains several Pautrier microabscesses. APAAP technique. (× 64)

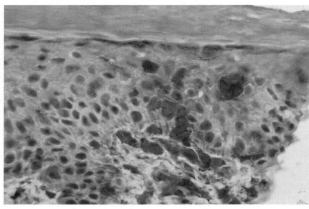

FIG. 30-42

Mycosis fungoides. Incubation with a monoclonal antibody against T helper cells (Leu 3a) shows Pautrier microabscesses in the epidermis. (× 160)

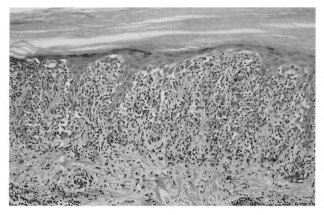

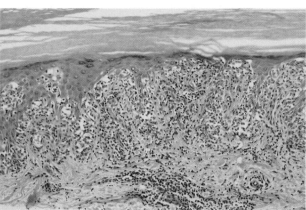

FIG. 30-43 and FIG. 30-44

Woringer-Kolopp disease. The epidermis is infiltrated by innumerable mononuclear cells. The infiltrating cells are surrounded by a halolike clear space. The dermis contains only a mild, nonspecific inflammatory infiltrate. (× 40)

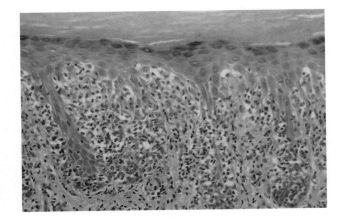

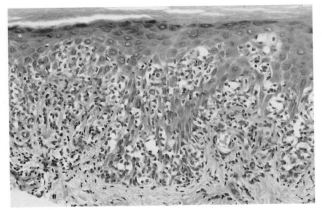

FIG. 30-45 and FIG. 30-46

Woringer-Kolopp disease. The lower portion of the epidermis is infiltrated by numerous mononuclear cells with hyperchromatic nuclei. The infiltrating cells have little cytoplasm and are surrounded by a halolike clear space. (× 64)

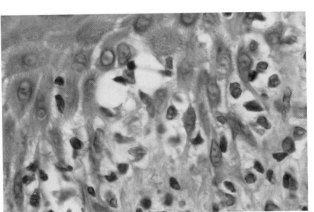

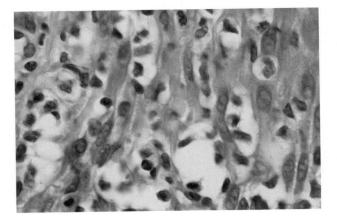

FIG. 30-47 and FIG. 30-48

Woringer-Kolopp disease. The infiltrating cells have convoluted hyperchromatic nuclei and are surrounded by a halolike clear space. (× 240)

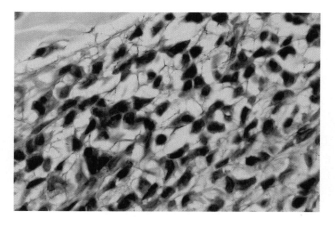

FIG. 30-49

Chronic granulocytic leukemia, Giemsa stain. The dermis is infiltrated by a dense cellular infiltrate. The cells have round, oval, or indented nuclei without recognizable granules. These cells are myelocytes and myeloblasts and are indistinguishable from immature cells seen in lymphoma. (× 240)

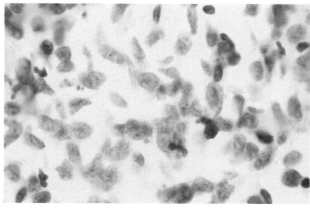

FIG. 30-50

Chronic granulocytic leukemia. Incubation with a polyclonal antibody against lysozyme reveals a positive reaction. This reaction is positive in myelocytes and myeloblasts. (× 240)

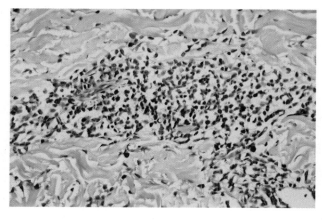

FIG. 30-51

Chronic granulocytic leukemia. Incubation with naphthol AS-D chloracetate esterase. Many of the infiltrate cells show a positive reaction. This reaction is positive in myelocytes and mature granulocytes but negative in myeloblasts. (× 64)

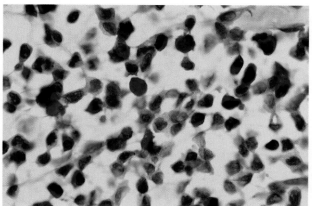

FIG. 30-52

Chronic granulocytic leukemia. Incubation with naphthol AS-D chloracetate esterase. The myelocytes show a positive reaction. (× 240)

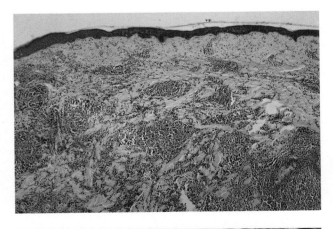

FIG. 30-53

Multiple myeloma. A dense infiltrate of atypical plasma cells is seen in the dermis. (× 16)

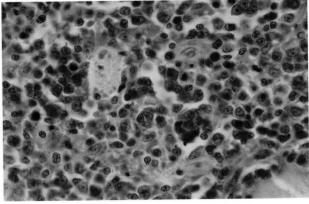

FIG. 30-54

Multiple myeloma. The plasma cells appear atypical and show variation in the size, shape, and staining intensity of the nuclei. (× 160)

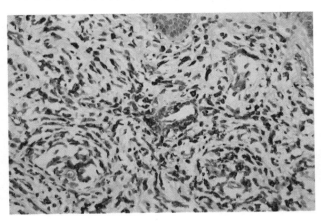

FIG. 30-55

Multiple myeloma. Incubation with a monoclonal antibody against lambda chains reveals a positive reaction in most cells. APAAP technique. (× 64)

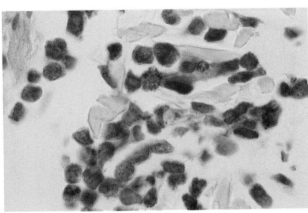

FIG. 30-56

Multiple myeloma. Incubation with a monoclonal antibody against lambda chains. Most plasma cells in this tumor contain lambda chains. A mitosis is present. APAAP technique. (× 240)

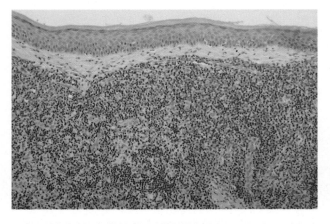

FIG. 30-57

Lympohocytoma cutis. The epidermis is flattened. The dermis contains a dense inflammatory infiltrate of lymphocytes that is separated from the overlying epidermis by a narrow grenz zone of normal collagen. (× 40)

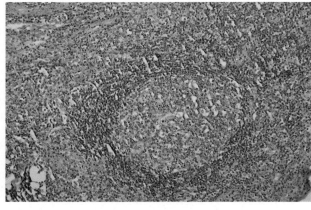

FIG. 30-58

Lymphocytoma cutis. The infiltrate consists of two types of cells arranged in this photomicrograph in a follicular pattern. The lighter-staining cells are follicular center cells. The small, dark-staining lymphocytes are T cells. (× 40)

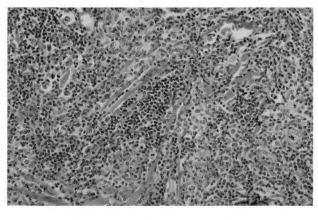

FIG. 30-59

Lymphocytoma cutis. The two types of cells are intermingled in this photomicrograph. The large, pale cells are macrophages. (× 64)

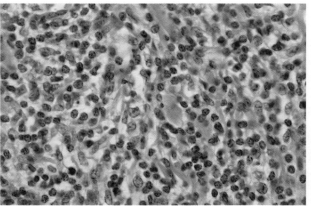

FIG. 30-60

Lymphocytoma cutis. The infiltrate consists of cells with small, dark nuclei and cells with large, pale-staining nuclei. (× 160)

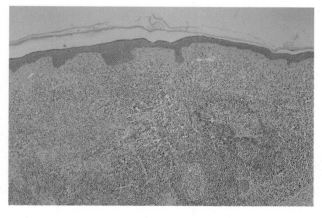

FIG. 30-61

Lymphocytoma cutis. The dermis contains a dense infiltrate that is separated from the epidermis by a narrow grenz zone of normal collagen. (× 16)

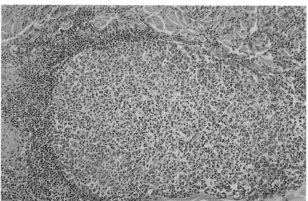

FIG. 30-62

Lymphocytoma cutis. The lesion consists of two types of cells in a follicular arrangement. The central, pale-staining cells are follicular center cells; the dark-staining cells are T cells. (× 40)

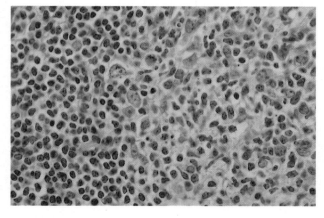

FIG. 30-63

Lymphocytoma cutis, higher magnification of the lymph follicle shown in Fig. 30-62. On the right side the majority of cells are pale-staining follicular center cells. The cells on the left side are T cells. (× 160)

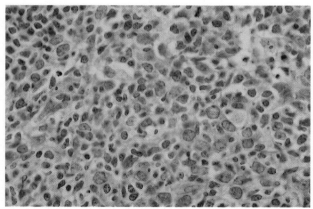

FIG. 30-64

Lymphocytoma cutis. The cells with dark-staining nuclei are intermingled with the cells with pale-staining nuclei. (× 160)

Index